AF344430

GENERAL SURGERY IN RELATION TO OBSTETRICS

Contemporary Surgical Management Series

- *Benign Diseases of the Esophagus:* Robert H. Quinn, M.D., John B. Gregg, M.D., and C. Douglas Wood, M.D.

- *Surgical Infections:* Edited by Lewis M. Flint, Jr., M.D., and Donald E. Fry, M.D.

- *Surgery of the Adrenal Glands:* Teruo Matsumoto, M.D., and A. Mohsen Kholoussy, M.D.

- *General Surgery in Relation to Obstetrics:* Edited by Neil R. Thomford, M.D.

GENERAL SURGERY IN RELATION TO OBSTETRICS

Contemporary Surgical Management

Edited by

Neil R. Thomford, M.D.
Professor and Chairman
Department of Surgery
Medical College of Ohio
Surgeon-in-Chief
Medical College of Ohio Hospital
Toledo, Ohio

MEDICAL EXAMINATION PUBLISHING CO., INC.
an Excerpta Medica company

Thomford, Neil R.
    General surgery in relation to obstetrics.

    (Contemporary surgical management series)
    Bibliography: p.
    Includes index.
    1. Surgery. 2. Pregnant women--Diseases. I. Title.
II. Series. [DNLM: 1. Pregnancy complications--Surgery.
2. Surgery, Operative--In pregnancy. WQ 400 G326]
RD31.5.T4 1984   618.3   83-26691
ISBN 0-87488-569-8

Printed in the United States of America

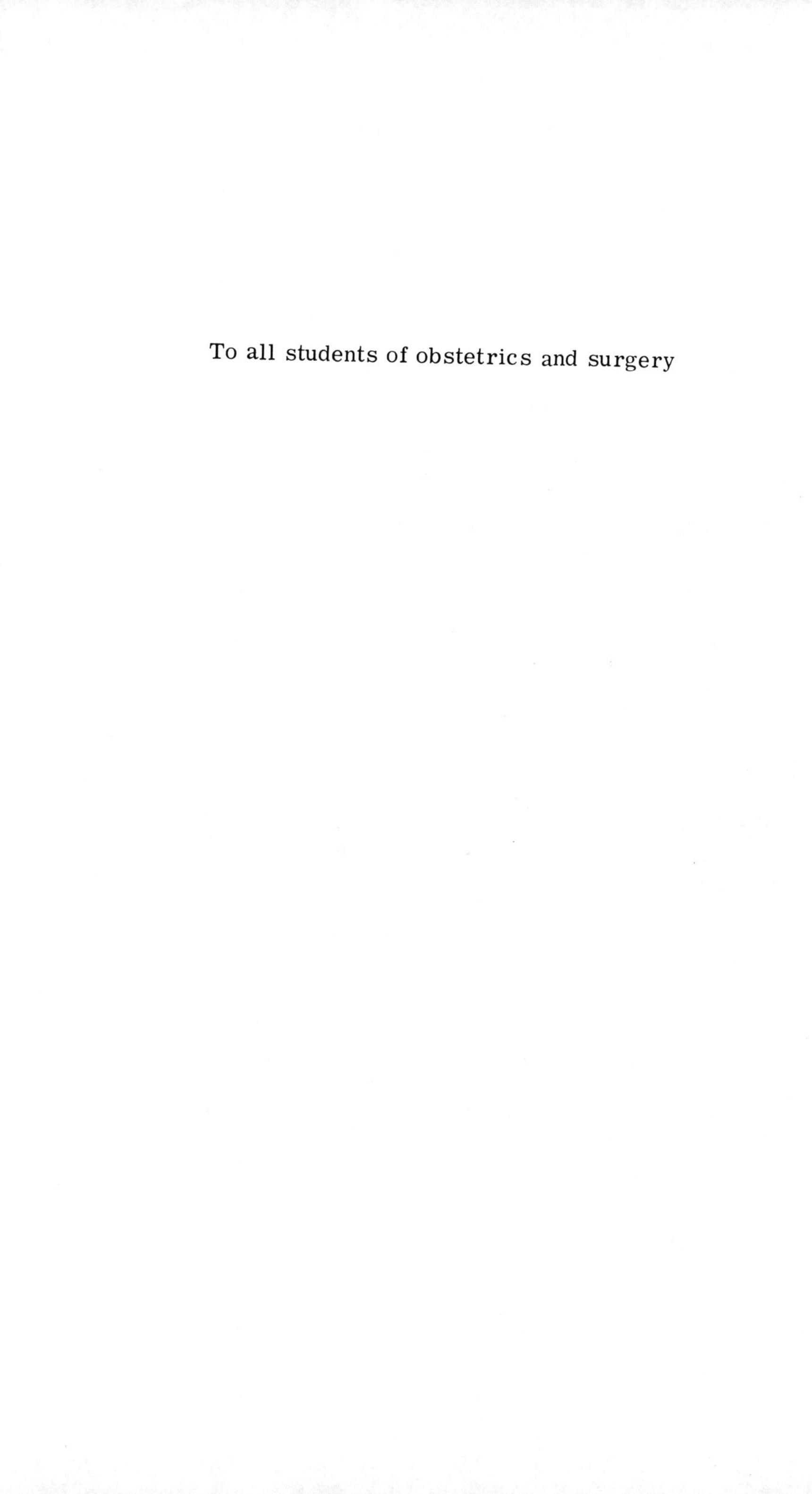

To all students of obstetrics and surgery

Contributors

DANIEL L. BROWN, Pharm.D., Clinical Pharmacist, Medical College of Ohio, Toledo

A. JOHN CHRISTOFORIDIS, M.D., Ph.D., Professor and Chairman, Department of Radiology, College of Medicine, Ohio State University, Columbus

JOHN TERRANCE DAVIS, M.D., Associate Professor of Surgery; Chief, Division of Cardio-Thoracic Surgery, Department of Surgery, Medical College of Ohio, Toledo

JOHN L. DUHRING, M.D., Faculty Chairman and Administrative Director, Department of Obstetrics and Gynecology, Medical College of Ohio, Toledo; Chairman, District V, American College of Obstetricians and Gynecologists

GEORGE P. GRECOS, M.D., Assistant Professor of Surgery, Medical College of Ohio, Toledo

JOHN T. MARTIN, M.D., Professor and Chairman, Department of Anesthesiology, Medical College of Ohio, Toledo

MELISSA A. MASH, M.D., Instructor and Chief Resident in Surgery, Medical College of Ohio, Toledo

HOLLIS W. MERRICK, M.D., M.Sc., F.A.C.S., F.R.C.S.(C), Associate Professor of Surgery, Medical College of Ohio, Toledo

J. ROBERT NAVARRE, M.D., F.A.C.S., Clinical Associate Professor of Surgery; Chief, Division of Peripheral Vascular Surgery, Department of Surgery, Medical College of Ohio, Toledo

JOE W. SAYRE, M.D., Resident in Surgery, Medical College of Ohio, Toledo

STEVEN H. SELMAN, M.D., Assistant Professor of Surgery (Urology), Medical College of Ohio, Toledo

PITAMBAR SOMANI, M.D., Ph.D., Director, Division of Clinical Pharmacology; Professor of Pharmacology and Medicine, Medical College of Ohio, Toledo

NEIL R. THOMFORD, M.D., Professor and Chairman, Department of Surgery, Medical College of Ohio; Surgeon-in-Chief, Medical College of Ohio Hospital, Toledo

ROBERT THOMPSON TIDRICK, M.D., F.A.C.S., Professor of Surgery, Medical College of Ohio, Toledo

Contents

Contributors   ix

Preface   xi

1   ANESTHETIC CONSIDERATIONS FOR SURGERY
DURING PREGNANCY   1
John T. Martin, M.D.

2   DIAGNOSTIC RADIOLOGICAL EXAMINATIONS
DURING PREGNANCY   12
A. John Christoforidis, M.D., Ph.D.

3   TRAUMA IN PREGNANCY   27
Joe W. Sayre, M.D., and
Neil R. Thomford, M.D.

4   ENDOCRINE DISORDERS   32
Melissa Mash, M.D.,
George P. Grecos, M.D., and
Neil R. Thomford, M.D.

5   GASTROINTESTINAL DISEASES DURING
PREGNANCY   43
George P. Grecos, M.D., and
Neil R. Thomford, M.D.

6   UROLOGIC PROBLEMS OF THE PREGNANT
PATIENT   67
Steven H. Selman, M.D.

7   PERIPHERAL VASCULAR PROBLEMS DURING
PREGNANCY   82
J. Robert Navarre, M.D.

viii / Contents

8   BREAST DISEASES DURING PREGNANCY   101
Robert T. Tidrick, M.D.

9   PREGNANCY AND CARDIOTHORACIC DISEASE   120
J. Terrance Davis, M.D.

10   THE MANAGEMENT OF HERNIAS DURING PREGNANCY   135
Hollis W. Merrick, M.D.

11   DRUG THERAPY DURING PREGNANCY   148
Pitambar Somani, M.D., Ph.D., and
Daniel Brown, Pharm.D.

12   OBSTETRICAL ADVANCES IN RELATION TO SURGICAL PRACTICE   180
John L. Duhring, M.D.

Index   185

Preface

This book is concerned with problems of the pregnant patient for which the general surgeon's assistance is often required. It is intended to serve as a text of selected fundamental knowledge for students of obstetrics and surgery, and as a current reference for practitioners of those disciplines.

Each contributor has reviewed a specific area and has provided cogent information regarding that subject. Of equal importance, however, are the more global reminders and messages for the reader. These include: 1) The clinical picture of most disease entities is much the same in the pregnant patient as in the nonpregnant patient; patient complaints must be carefully assessed and not casually attributed to a normal intrauterine pregnancy. 2) The risk-benefit equation for most diagnostic tests is such that if there is proper indication for the examination it should in most instances be done even though the patient is pregnant; physicians should not place their patients at a disadvantage as a result of the general reluctance to obtain diagnostic studies when a patient is pregnant. 3) Operations may be done with relative safety during pregnancy; this is particularly true today with the availability of medication to limit the risk of onset of labor after operation.

We hope those who practice obstetrics and those surgeons who see pregnant patients in consultation will include this book in their working library. If so, our goal of increasing the safety of pregnancy for the mother and the unborn child will by some measure be realized.

The response and cooperation of the contributing authors was excellent. I am grateful to each of them and to my administrative assistant, Ms. Judy Fegley, for her invaluable assistance in bringing the project to fruition.

notice

The editor and authors and the publisher of this book have
made every effort to ensure that all therapeutic modalities that
are recommended are in accordance with accepted standards
at the time of publication.

The drugs specified within this book may not have specific
approval from the Food and Drug Administration in regard to
the indications and dosages that may be recommended by the
authors. The manufacturer's package insert is the best source
of current prescribing information.

Chapter 1

ANESTHETIC CONSIDERATIONS FOR SURGERY DURING PREGNANCY

John T. Martin, M.D.

Estimates of the number of pregnant women who are anesthetized for purposes other than obstetrical delivery vary from 0.3 to 2.2% of all pregnancies and represent about 50,000 patients annually in the United States. (1, 2) Basic concerns of the anesthesiologist regarding this patient population relate to three major issues: (1) recognizing the physiologic alterations produced by the pregnancy and avoiding maternal complications, (2) minimizing insults to the fetus, and (3) avoiding stimulation of premature labor. But the ultimate concern has to do with the possibility that anesthesia may cause maldevelopment or death of the fetus or maturational problems to be displayed later by the infant. We will examine these concerns in light of recent data.

PERTINENT MATERNAL PHYSIOLOGY

The respiratory system of the mother changes in important ways as pregnancy progresses. The diaphragm is forced cephalad by the enlarging uterus and compensatory changes occur in the antero-posterior diameter of the thorax as well as in the lateral expansion. Inspiratory capacity and inspiratory reserve volume are increased, while expiratory reserve volume, residual volume, and functional residual capacity (FRC) all decrease. On the balance, total lung capacity is unchanged. Progesterone-induced bronchodilation occurs, and the mucosa of the respiratory tract becomes congested, easily friable, and susceptible to mechanical injury from suction catheters and endotracheal tubes. Ventilation increases early in pregnancy and remains elevated to term. Tidal volume is increased by 40%, respiratory rate by 15%, and minute ventilation by 50% at term. (3) Because dead space is unchanged, net alveolar ventilation is about 70% greater than in the nonpregnant patient. The resulting chronic hypocapnea ($PaCO_2$ 32-33 torr) is matched by renal losses of fixed base to retain arterial pH within normal limits. An increased basal metabolic rate (BMR) and, perhaps, an impaired diffusion of oxygen across the pulmonary membrane(4) necessitate the ventilatory increase. The FRC decrease lessens pulmonary oxygen content and implies an earlier onset of hypoxia in the presence of either respiratory obstruction or the prolonged apnea that may occur during a difficult endotracheal intubation. Increased alveolar ventilation hastens uptake of an inhaled anesthetic agent, shortens induction time, and may undesirably increase tissue concentrations of the anesthetic unless the effects are carefully monitored.

Important <u>cardiovascular</u> changes begin early in pregnancy and increase variably to term. Cardiac output and stroke volume are increased 30-50%(5), and blood volume increases 25-40% by the second trimester because of the additional perfusion requirements of the developing placenta and fetus. Systemic vascular resistance decreases (including uterine vascular resistance), heart rate rises somewhat, and the net effect on blood pressure is usually a modest decrease. As the uterus enlarges, with the patient supine, blood return via the inferior vena cava is increasingly obstructed and diverts into the vertebral and peridural plexuses and thence into the superior vena cava via the azygos system. (6) The resulting engorgement of epidural and subarachnoid vessels reduces the size of the cerebrospinal fluid spaces in the spine and is traditionally thought to augment cephalad spread of the subarachnoid or epidural dose of a conduction anesthetic agent. (2) However, Grundy and colleagues, (7) in a study of epidural anesthesia in humans, have been unable to substantiate this assumption.

Howard et al. (8) first described a syncopal syndrome in pregnant women who were supine. They reported that about 10% showed hypotension, tachycardia, pallor, and faintness due to the cava being compressed by the uterine mass late in pregnancy. Recent data have indicated an increase in the incidence to 90%, recognized an earlier onset, and shown that the aorta is compressed as well. Accordingly, the situation is more properly referred to as "aorto-caval compression" rather than the original description, "supine hypotensive syndrome."(6) Uteroplacental and renal flow are reduced in the supine patient and restored when the patient is tilted toward the left flank to relieve the compression (so-called "left uterine displacement").

While blood volume increases by about 40% over normal at term, red blood cell mass increases less (20%) than does plasma volume (50%) with the result that decreased laboratory values of hemoglobin, red cell count, and hematocrit might be misunderstood as "anemia." Hemoglobin values below 10 g/dl and hematocrits below 30% should be viewed as abnormal, but the usual gestational hypervolemia amounts to a gain of 1200-1500 ml of volume and permits an appreciable blood loss prior to necessary replacements.

Platelets increase to over 300,000/mm^3 at term, fibrinogen content rises from 250 to 450 mg/dl, and blood clotting factors increase. The term patient, then, is apt to be on the borderline of hypercoagulability and hence to be susceptible to thromboembolic complications. (9)

Serum cholinesterase levels fall by 20% early in pregnancy. Nevertheless, the enzyme remains structurally unaltered and seems to be functionally sufficient to permit use of "normal" (50-400 mg) amounts of succinylcholine for maternal intubation and muscle relaxation. (10)

The changes in the upper gastrointestinal tract of the pregnant patient can be a threat to her safety. As the uterus enlarges it displaces the stomach in a horizontal manner with the cephalad and dorsal shift of the pylorus prolonging gastric emptying(5) by as much as 60%. Pain, anxiety, and drug administration further lengthen emptying time. Intragastric pressure increases toward term as does the tone of the lower esophageal sphincter.(11) Women who have heartburn have been found to have a loose lower esophageal sphincter, which permits reflux of acid gastric contents into the esophagus and increases the risk of regurgitation and aspiration.

Drugs which increase intragastric or intra-abdominal pressure or relax the lower esophageal sphincter promote regurgitation. Those which tighten the sphincter, shorten gastric transit time, and promote pyloric relaxation reduce the opportunity for regurgitation. Fasciculations produced by intravenous doses of succinylcholine increase abdominal muscle tone and, thereby, compress the stomach to raise intragastric pressure. Prior administration of 3-6 mg curare by slow injection (or infusion) or succinylcholine will minimize or abolish the intragastric pressure rise. Atropine premedication reduces lower esophageal sphincter tone. Dopamine has also been found to relax the sphincter. Metoclopramide increases lower esophageal sphincter tone, increases gastric peristalsis, shortens gastric transit time, relaxes the pyloric sphincter, and promotes gastric emptying, apparently without increasing either gastric secretion or gastric acidity. Domperidone, an anti-emetic, blocks dopamine receptors and increases lower esophageal sphincter tone. Dow and Brock-Utne (12, 13) in South Africa have demonstrated the relaxant effect of atropine on the lower esophageal sphincter and have advocated adding either metoclopramide or domperidone to the pre-anesthetic drug regimen to protect against gastric reflux, regurgitation, and aspiration.

Reducing the volume of gastric secretions and raising gastric pH above 2.5 also are methods of protection against aspiration pneumonitis. Antacids have been used prior to anesthesia to raise gastric pH. Particulate antacids control pH but, if aspirated, produce lasting bronchopneumonia, hypoxia, and fibrosis. (14) Sodium citrate, also an effective antacid, is not particulate and, thus, is not as injurious to the lung if aspirated. However, it is unpleasant to take, increases gastric fluid volume, and does not suppress gastric secretion. (15) Cimetidine is a histamine receptor blocker and decreases gastric acid secretion. Dundee reported 40 patients for caesarean section who received cimetidine 400 mg orally before anesthesia in whom gastric pH rose to levels above 2.5 when sampled 1 to 2-$\frac{1}{2}$ hours postadministration. (16)

FETAL CONSIDERATIONS

Chronic exposure of pregnant women to the operating room environment has been shown to increase the incidence of spontaneous abortions and congenital abnormalities in their offspring when compared to offspring of women without operating room association. (17) A similar relationship has been shown for indirect exposure, namely, pregnancies of nonoperating room women impregnated by males who work in the operating room. Whether environmental stress is the hazard or the increased incidence represents the effects of prolonged exposure to trace concentrations of anesthetic gases and vapors is currently undecided. (18) Hopefully, the installation and evaluation of competent systems for scavenging traces of anesthetic gases in the operating rooms will help clarify the issue in the near future.

Teratogenicity can be shown to be produced in laboratory animals by acute exposure of fetuses to a large number of anesthetic and nonanesthetic drugs. (5) Ill effects vary with the drug used, the time during fetal organogenesis at which exposure occurs, and the sensitivity of the animal species involved. Extreme species differences preclude extrapolation of available animal data to humans, Three human studies have suggested an association between minor tranquilizers used by the mother during pregnancy and congenital malformations of the offspring.

(19, 20, 21) However, a fourth study(22) involving 50,000 human pregnancies failed to support these findings. While the data are not conclusive, the FDA has cautioned against the use of minor tranquilizers in the first trimester of pregnancy.

Hyperbaric oxygen is known to be teratogenic in animals, but high concentrations of oxygen at normal atmospheric pressure is not. No evidence exists that brief exposure to hypoxia, hypo-cardia, or hypercarbia is teratogenic in humans despite isolated anecdotal assertions. Chronic hypoxemia of high altitude of living is not teratogenic. (2)

Widespread allegations, apparently based upon improper interpretations of data, hold that even conventional doses of medications or anesthetics administered during delivery may produce permanent central nervous system dysfunction in offspring. (23) Careful studies now underway in medical centers do not support these allegations. At present there is no evidence that anesthesia administered to a pregnant women adversely affects later mental or neurologic development of the infant (so-called "behavioral teratology"). (24) No anesthetic agents have been shown to be carcinogenic. (25)

Intrauterine fetal asphyxia, an issue of major importance, is avoided by maintaining normal maternal PaO_2, $PaCO_2$, and uterine perfusion.

Maternal hypoxia occurs as the result of laryngeal spasm, airway obstruction, adverse endotracheal tube positioning, and/or inadequate inspired oxygen concentration as well as from ventilatory depression due either to excessive concentrations of general anesthetic agents or to high somatic levels of spinal or epidural anesthesia. Increasing maternal oxygenation increases fetal oxygenation; no studies have shown uteroplacental vasoconstriction in vivo or fetal hypoxia following maternal hyperoxia. (26) Because of high oxygen consumption of the placenta and its uneven distribution of maternal and fetal blood flow, fetal PaO_2 levels high enough to close the ductus arteriosus or produce retrolental fibroplasia do not occur in utero. With maternal PaO_2 as high as 600 torr, fetal PaO_2 does not exceed 60 torr. (2)

Alterations in maternal $PaCO_2$ have a direct effect upon the fetus. Maternal hypocarbia causes vasoconstriction of placental vessels. In addition, alkalosis shifts the oxyhemoglobin dissociation curve to the left and less oxygen is available at the placenta. Fetal hypoxia results, and fetal acidosis follows. Increased maternal $PaCO_2$ is directly reflected in fetal acidosis.

Maternal hypotension threatens uterine blood flow unless uterine vascular resistance also is decreased. (2) Reduced uterine blood flow produces fetal asphyxia, fetal brain damage, fetal myocardial failure, and fetal death. The magnitude of the effect depends upon the degree and duration of the perfusion deficit. Increased uterine vascular resistance may also impair uterine blood flow. Uterine hypertonus, endogenous sympathetic discharge, use of alpha-adrenergic vasopressors, and systemic uptake of epinephrine from regional block solutions all have been implicated as uterine vasoconstrictors. Ketamine in excess of about 1. 0 mg/kg(27) is a uterine vasoconstrictor as are toxic doses of conduction agents.

Should maternal hypotension occur during regional or general anesthesia, prompt correction is mandatory. The critical level of maternal systolic pressure has been described as (1) a 25-30% decrease below its pre-anesthetic measurement or (2) less than 100 torr if the pre-anesthetic value exceeds 100 torr with the mother on her side to obviate aorto-caval compression. (28) Treatment includes eliminating aortocaval compression by lateral uterine displacement, minimizing the concentration of the inhalation agent, rapidly infusing crystalloid solutions if vasodilation has occurred with regional anesthesia, replacing significant amounts of shed blood, and, last, judiciously using a vasopressor. Ephedrine and mephentermine both act primarily by increasing cardiac output and will raise maternal pressure (assuming adequate volume and caval return) with the least amount of uterine vasoconstriction and the least additional interference with fetal perfusion. Those vasopressors which act principally by constricting the peripheral vasculature may elevate maternal pressure, vasoconstrict placental vessels, and not improve fetal perfusion. (28)

PREMATURE DELIVERY AND PERINATAL MORTALITY

Shnider and Webster reported a series of 9073 patients who delivered infants at the University of California Medical Center, San Francisco, between 1959 and 1964. (10) One hundred forty-seven had surgical procedures while pregnant. Premature delivery occurring within two weeks after operation was considered to be potentially influenced by anesthesia, the operative procedure, or the condition requiring the surgery. Three premature deliveries (6. 4%) took place in the 47 patients having surgery in the first trimester of gestation, five out of 58 (8. 5%) in the second trimester, and five out of 42 (11. 9%) in the third trimester. Roughly, this represents one episode of premature labor per twelve patients.

The anesthetic agent or technique played no role in premature labor; however, the type of operation was significant. While the overall premature delivery rate in the University of California series was 8. 8%, that following Shirodkar procedures for repair of an incomplete cervix was 28% and was associated with a 33% fetal mortality. Smith(29) reported 40% premature deliveries in his Shirodkar series, and all fetuses perished.

Among patients whose pregnancy did not include a surgical procedure the perinatal mortality rate was 2. 1%; for those who underwent surgery, 7. 5%. However, if the group of patients for Shirodkar procedures is excluded from the surgical series the perinatal mortality was 3. 8%, a figure that is not statistically different from the nonsurgical group.

Little additional information exists about the role of anesthetics in stimulating or inhibiting the onset of premature delivery. Prudence would seem to suggest avoiding ketamine in doses over 1. 1 mg/kg, avoiding uterotonic vasopressors, and slowly injecting cholinergic drugs that might produce uterine hypertonicity. But firm data are lacking. (2)

ANESTHETIC MANAGEMENT

Levinson and Shnider(2) have made specific recommendations for the anesthetic management of pregnant patients:

1. Elective surgery should be postponed until after delivery.

2. Although no drug associated with anesthesia has been proven teratogenic in humans, fetal exposure during organogenesis (the first trimester) should be avoided whenever possible and urgent surgery should be delayed until the second or third trimester.

3. Emergency surgery should employ regional anesthesia whenever feasible. Spinal anesthesia minimizes fetal exposure to local anesthetic agents.

4. The pre-anesthetic visit should be used to attempt to allay maternal apprehension. Barbiturates are preferable to minor tranquilizer as sedatives. Glycopyrrolate is an anticholinergic agent that does not cross the placenta.

5. No one technique of general anesthesia has been found to be superior. Usage has shown thiopental, succinylcholine, curare, morphine, meperidine, nitrous oxide, and halothane to be safe. Adequate maternal oxygenation and avoidance of hyperventilation during general anesthesia are mandatory.

6. Prevention of aspiration pneumonitis with antacids, cricoid pressure, endotracheal intubation (general anesthesia), etc. is important and should be routine.

7. The left lateral tilt posture to minimize aortocaval compression should be used in the second and third trimester.

8. Continuous fetal heart rate monitoring should accompany surgery after the sixteenth week of pregnancy. Postoperatively the uterine activity should be continuously monitored to detect the onset of premature labor. Betamimetic therapy may prevent preterm delivery.

Based upon these evaluations of available evidence we may reasonably conclude that anesthetic agents by themselves have not been found to be either carcinogenic or teratogenic in humans, that they bear no clear responsibility for causing premature labor, and that subsequent behavioral abnormalities in the neonate which have been ascribed to anesthetics are not substantiated. With careful understanding of the changes in maternal physiology which accompany pregnancy and of the unique characteristics of the utero-placental-fetal interrelationships, anesthesia without undue risk to mother and fetus can be offered to the woman who requires a surgical procedure for reasons unrelated to her pregnancy.

REFERENCES

1. Brodsky, JB, et al. Surgery during pregnancy and fetal outcome. Am. J. Obstet. Gynecol., 138:1165-1167, 1980.

2. Shnider, SM, and Levinson, G. Anesthesia for Obstetrics. Baltimore, MD, Williams and Wilkins, 1979, pp. 312-330.

3. Anderson, GJ, James, GB, Mathers, NP, et al. The maternal oxygen tension and acid-base status during pregnancy. J. Obstet. Gynecol. Br. Commonw., 76:16-19, 1969.

4. Dick, W, Ahnfeld, FW, Milewski, P, et al. Important clinical adaptation processes of women during pregnancy: Anesthesiologic considerations. J. Perinat. Med., 5:103-113, 1977.

5. Pederson, H, and Finster, J. Anesthetic risk in the pregnant surgical patient. Anesthesiol. 51:439-451, 1979.

6. Kerr, MG, Scott, DB, and Samuel, E. Studies of the inferior vena cava in late pregnancy. Br. Med. J., 1:532-533, 1964.

7. Grundy, EM, Zamora, AM, and Winnie, AP. Comparison of spread of epidural anesthesia in pregnant and nonpregnant women. Anesth. Analg., 57:544-546, 1978.

8. Howard, BK, Goodson, JH, and Mengert, WF. Supine hypotensive syndrome of late pregnancy. Obstet. Gynecol., 1:381-387, 1953.

9. Marx, GF, and Orkin, LR. Physiology of Obstetric Anesthesia. Springfield, Ill., Charles C Thomas, 1969, p. 18.

10. Shnider, SM. Serum cholinesterase activity during pregnancy, labor and the puerpeium. Anesthesiol., 26:335-339, 1965.

11. Lind, FJ, Smith, AM, Melver, DK, et al. Heartburn in pregnancy — A manometric study. Can. Med. Assoc. J., 98:571, 1968.

12. Down, TGB, et al. Effect of atropine on lower esophageal sphincter in late pregnancy. Obstet. Gynecol., 51:426-430, 1978.

13. Brock-Utne, JG, et al. Effect of domperidone on lower esophageal sphincter in late pregnancy. Anesthesiol., 52:321-323, 1980.

14. Gibbs, CP, et al. Antacid pulmonary aspiration in the dog. Anesthesiol., 51:380-385, 1979.

15. Gibbs, CP, et al. In vitro and in vivo evaluation of sodium citrate as an antacid. Anesthesiol., 55:A311, 1981.

16. Dundee, JW, et al. Use of cimetidine as an oral antacid in obstetric anesthesia. Anesth. Analg. (Abstr.), 60:246-247, 1981.

17. Spence, AA, Cohen, EN, Brown, BW, Jr., et al. Occupational hazards for operating room-based physicians: Analyses of data from the United States and the United Kingdom. JAMA, 238:321, 1974.

18. Cohen, EN, Brown, BW, Bruse, DL, et al. Occupational disease among operating room personnel: A national study. Anesthesiol., 41:321, 1974.

19. Milkovich, L, and van den Bert, BJ. Effects of prenatal meprobamate and chlordiazepoxide hydrochloride on human embryonic and fetal development. N. Engl. J. Med., 291:1268, 1974.

20. Saxen, I, and Saxen, L. Association between maternal intake of diazepam and oral clefts. Lancet, 2:498, 1975.

21. Safra, MJ, and Oakley, GP. Association between cleft lip with or without cleft palate and prenatal exposure to diazepam. Lancet, 2:478, 1975.

22. Hartz, SC, Heinomen, OP, Shapiro, S, et al. Antenatal exposure to meprobamate and chlordiazepoxide in relation to malformations, mental development, and childhood mortality. N. Engl. J. Med., 292:726, 1965.

23. Kolata, GB. Behavioral teratology: Birth defects of the mind. Science, 101:732, 1978.

24. Committee on Drugs of the American Academy of Pediatrics and the Committee on Obstetrics: Maternal and Fetal Medicine of the American College of Obstetrics and Gynecologists: Effect of medication during labor and delivery on infant outcome. Pediatrics, 62:402, 1978.

25. Eger, EL II, White, AE, and Brown, CL. A test of carcinogenicity of enflurane, isoflurane, halothane, methoxyflurane, and nitrous oxide in mice. Anesth. Analg. 57:678, 1978.

26. Khazin, AF, Hon, EH, and Hehre, FW. Effects of maternal hyperoxia on the fetus. I. Oxygen tension. Am. J. Obstet. Gynecol., 109:628, 1971.

27. Galloon, S. Ketamine for obstetric delivery. Anesthesiol., 44:522, 1976.

28. Gutsche, BB. Prevention of hypotension during regional anesthesia: <u>Abstract in Obstetrical Anesthesia,</u> State of the Art, Course Syllabus, Shnider, SM, and Levinson, G, eds. University of California at San Francisco Medical Center, 1982.

29. Smith, BE. Fetal prognosis after anesthesia during gestation. <u>Anesth. Analg.</u>, 42:521, 1963.

Chapter 2

DIAGNOSTIC RADIOLOGICAL EXAMINATIONS
DURING PREGNANCY

A. John Christoforidis, M. D.,

INTRODUCTION

The spectrum of radiological diagnostic procedures used today involves primarily ionizing radiation. Other forms of energy used include ultrasound waves and recently nuclear magnetic
resonance which do not possess the property of ionization. The
lack of ionization encourages the use of ultrasound for the examination of the pregnant woman. Routine radiological diagnostic
examinations such as the chest x-ray and examinations of the
gastrointestinal tract, of the skeleton, of the urinary tract, and
of the circulatory system and all the invasive radiological procedures should be available to the pregnant woman as to any
other patient. Her unique physiological status, however, requires special consideration and imposes some restrictions,
particularly because of the fetus she is carrying.

Therefore, in recommending or performing any radiological
procedures on pregnant women, one should always take into
consideration not only the woman but also keep in mind the possibility of radiation exposure of the unborn embryo-fetus. The
axiom _primum non lacerare_ (do not harm) always should be a
guide in medical practice and especially should be in our minds
when considering a diagnostic examination for the pregnant
woman.

The referring physician should have a basic background
knowledge regarding the exposure doses to the embryo-fetus and
the acceptable limits of exposure levels for which no injurious
effects of ionizing radiation are known. The physician should
have a record of the patient and ask about any previous examinations with ionizing radiation during the same pregnancy.
Under these conditions the responsible physician is aware of

the amount of radiation received by the embryo-fetus so that the total exposure will be kept within low and acceptable limits. The physician should remember that when an examination is indicated the pregnant woman should have the benefit of the diagnostic examination, which in many cases cannot be postponed until the termination of her pregnancy.

The performance of a needed examination may not only be vital for the expectant mother's health but also for her fetus, the well-being of which is obviously dependent upon her condition. Of course no patient should be submitted to an examination unless there are indications for it and therefore benefits to be derived. While this principle for the examination of any patient should not be violated, in the case of the pregnant patient this becomes of utmost importance. Once this principle is understood and followed carefully, then the woman should not be deprived of the benefits of proper patient care which include the necessary diagnostic studies.

This brief chapter particularly addresses the important issue of radiation exposure with the objective of giving the reader some pertinent basic information. It is not unusual for an inadequately informed physician to ask for an unnecessary and potentially hazardous examination. In other instances the pregnant patient may be deprived of a vital and safe examination (such as a chest examination) because the physician again has inadequate information and believes the study to have hazards for the embryo-fetus or the mother. By being better informed the physician also can discuss further specific problems with the radiologist and then explain them to the patient and answer possible questions. A significant number of patients today are informed (not always correctly) about radiation hazards from different public information media, without the necessary background for an accurate and in-depth understanding of the problem.

Radiation-induced hazards have been known since the early days of its medical use. It is worth mentioning that cases of radiation injury were reported a short time following the discovery of the roentgen rays in 1895 in the form of acute radiation injuries due to large exposure to ionizing radiation. As early as 1902 we can find reports of carcinoma induced by ionizing radiation. It was several years later that the significance of exposure to relatively low doses of radiation and their biological effects were appreciated. An in-depth study of the effects of ionizing radiation started after World War II as a result of the historic impact of the explosions of two atomic bombs.

The thousands of survivors covering the spectrum of all ages and including a significant number of pregnant women were carefully scrutinized, studied, and followed. (12, 20) Their children and grandchildren are still being studied carefully. The moral obligation to help the victims of that horrifying experience and the worldwide interest in getting answers to many questions related to the biological effects of ionizing radiation in humans gave much support to these studies. The catastrophic results of the atomic explosions in Hiroshima and Nagasaki, ironically, thus became a source from which knowledge has been derived for the benefit of surviving humans. (11)

There has been an increasing number of scientific papers dealing with the hazards or potential hazards of ionizing radiation and particularly the radiation used for medical diagnostic purposes. The ever-increasing interest and justifiable concern of the physicians as well as of the informed public stimulated further research and increased the body of our knowledge. We are presenting here the information known to us currently and are emphasizing the facts related to diagnostic radiological procedures for pregnant or for potentially pregnant women and the possible hazards.

The significance and the magnitude of this problem is reflected by the large amount of publicity on this subject by the public media. In addition, scientific societies and particularly the medical ones as well as the U.S. Department of Health, Education, and Welfare have become involved not only in providing the correct information to the public and to the users of ionizing radiation but also in legislating and enforcing the guidelines according to our present scientific knowledge.

DIAGNOSTIC RADIOLOGICAL EXAMINATIONS AND RADIATION EXPOSURE

As background information, it is of interest to mention that in 1978 the total number of radiographic examinations reached approximately 130 million out of which 65.2 million involved the thorax, 32.0 million involved the abdomen, 22.0 million involved the extremities, and 10 million involved the head, neck, and other parts of the body. The total number of fluoroscopic examinations was approximately 12.0 million, out of which 6.6 million were gastrointestinal series, 3.5 million involved barium enemas, and all the other fluoroscopic examinations amounted to approximately 2.0 million. However, the number of pregnant women involved in these examinations is not known exactly.

Our interest here is focused on the exposure levels as related to the uterus or embryo-fetus during the diagnostic procedures. Table 2-1 gives the estimated dose to the ovaries and uterus in

Table 2-1: Estimated dose to the ovaries (uterus) expressed in millirads per radiographic examination.

Type of Examination	Estimated Dose
Chest radiograph	1
Mammography	10
Upper GI series	171
Cholecystography	78
Extremities	0.5
Thoracic spine	11
Lumbar spine	400
Pelvis	250
IVP (urography)	588
Barium enema	903

millirads of commonly performed radiographic examinations. The information in this table is taken from a report by the National Council on Radiation Protection and Measurements (NCRP), No. 54, 1977.

It should be pointed out that there is a significant variation of the above numbers, depending upon several factors which include the collimation and also the filtration of the x-ray beam, the kilovoltage and the milliamperes used, the distance from the x-ray tube to the part of the body examined, the size of the field used, and the number of radiographs obtained during the examination. In case of fluoroscopic examination, the time of fluoroscopy and the number and size of the fluoroscopic spot films should be taken into consideration when estimating the total amount of radiation exposure delivered to the uterus. The numbers in Table 2-1 are not intended to tell us the exact amount of radiation received by a specific patient but rather to give us a general and yet realistic background knowledge of the approximate amount of radiation to which the embryo-fetus is exposed during the performance of the more common diagnostic procedures.

There is significant evidence indicating that the amount of ionizing radiation to which the embryo-fetus is exposed can damage a human being. This has been demonstrated in a number of different ways primarily in experimental animals but also in humans. Retrospective studies of humans exposed in utero, while their mothers were examined for diagnostic purposes or during the time when radiation treatments were considered acceptable for benign conditions, have been conducted for many years. The exposure of pregnant women at the time of the atomic explosions at the conclusion of World War II who subsequently delivered were also studied in great detail.

It should be stated that today indications for the examination of pregnant patients involve only diagnostic procedures. During these examinations, the amount of ionizing radiation used is a small fraction of the amount utilized during the x-ray examination on which the above-mentioned studies were based. The reason for this becomes obvious when one considers the present regulations for manufacturing x-ray equipment, the carefully observed restrictions in their utilization, and the mandatory educational requirements for all the personnel licensed to use the equipment. These regulations did not exist in earlier years.

The diagnostic procedures might be related to the pregnancy of the woman. More often, however, they are not directly related to her pregnancy and yet are very important to the well-being of the embryo-fetus she is carrying.

RADIATION HAZARDS

The vital element involved in the process of ionization, with potentially hazardous effects, is the nucleus of the cell. The transfer of energy taking place is related to the amount of radiation acting upon the nucleus. In the case where the amount of radiation used is large enough, the cell may be destroyed. When the amount of energy transferred to the nucleus is relatively low, then the deleterious effects depend upon the degree of injury, which varies according to the amount of radiation absorbed. One of the most important considerations during the cellular damage is the precipitation of potentially malignant changes to the cellular population of the embryo-fetus.

It is logical to consider that if the cells involved in this process are part of the hemopoietic system then, depending on the precursor cell or cells, a form of leukemia might develop. If the injury involves the precursor cells of an organ, then a defective development of that particular organ will result. The present literature contains several reports supporting the thesis that diagnostic radiological procedures have precipitated a statistically significant increase in leukemia particularly during childhood. (3, 4, 5, 7, 8, 9,) However, there is disagreement among the investigators regarding the exact number of childhood leukemia cases expected, above and beyond the anticipated number of cases of the disease in the general population. It is generally accepted that there is a proportional relationship between prenatal radiation exposure and leukemia. (22) The relationship between leukemia and the amount of radiation causing this disease during life is probably linear, with the increase of the incidence of leukemia being proportional to the dosage of radiation to which the fetus has been exposed. In the nonexposed population, the estimated incidence of leukemia among whites is 1 in 2880 children below the age of 10 years.

It has been postulated, based on statistics which include experimental data, that when children are exposed in utero in the first trimester to the level of 2000 mrad (2 rad) leukemia occurs in the ratio of 1 in 2000 cases below the age of 10. This is a risk factor for this level of radiation exposure in relation to the population of pregnant women not submitted to any radiation (except to the unavoidable cosmic radiation which is part of our living environment).

While there is a relationship between prenatal radiation and a statistically demonstrable increase in leukemia, this has not been the case with the incidence of solid tumors. (23, 24, 25) This is much more difficult to study statistically for at least two important reasons. The first is the broad spectrum of the different types of solid tumors and their different behavior. The second is the fact that the manifestations and development of solid tumors occur later in life, and therefore the tracing of these patients 40 or 50 years later is very difficult. Their mothers' record so many years later is usually lost or difficult to obtain. In the case of childhood leukemia under the age of 10, the collection of statistical data is obviously much easier to follow and therefore more reliable.

There is general acceptance, as mentioned above, that exposure of the fetus to 2000 mrad of radiation has as a result the increase of the possibility of developing leukemia from 1 in 2880 cases, in the nonradiated population, to 1 in 2000. Therefore, the critical question raised is: Should the physician advise interruption of pregnancy in the case of a pregnant woman exposed to 2 rad in the region of her uterus ? This dilemma is very difficult to solve, because the answer should take into consideration other important factors which differ from one patient to another.

Let us think of the pregnant woman who has had a child who developed leukemia and is pregnant again. Without any irradiation the chances of the sibling developing leukemia, according to reliable statistical data, is not 1 in 2880 (nonradiated population) but 1 in 720. (22) It is very difficult to believe that this expectant mother will interrupt her pregnancy in spite of the fact that the risk factor is relatively higher (almost three times) in comparison with the woman who does not have this history but whose fetus received **2000 mrad** in the process of a diagnostic examination. Even so, a chance of 1 in 720 is not really very significant.

I believe that these comparative and scientifically acceptable figures can give us a more realistic and humane approach to a very serious problem where the physician has the obligation to advise and the woman and the father the right to decide. Obviously other very important factors will have to be taken into consideration, including her age and religious and ethnic background, the possible hazards to the life of the expectant mother from the abortion, the laws of the state as related to the legality of the abortion, and of course the presence of other children in the family. For the woman who was not fortunate enough to have conceived previously to accept a small risk for her unborn child might be more reasonable and acceptable. It is a decision which only she and her family can make and live with after being properly informed by a physician who is familiar with the known scientific facts.

The physician who recommends the radiological examination should be guided by certain rules which are generally accepted and outlined in the NCRP's (National Council on Radiation Protection and Measurements) Report No. 54. During the preimplantation stage (this includes the first ten days of pregnancy), an exposure of the uterus to above 10 rad (10,000 mrad) will have an effect which might not be leukemogenic or carcinogenic but will increase the incidence of intrauterine death. At the preimplantation stage the cells are not yet differentiated and have the potential to replace other also undifferentiated cells without producing defects in future organs. If the number of cells killed is large, then an early abortion (which might not even be noticed) will take place. As the pregnancy progresses and implantation occurs the differentiation of the cells and the organogenesis starts. Here the loss of a few cells, which by now are differentiated, is not fatal, but the organ which will result from these cells might become defective. This possibility increases when the fetus is exposed to 25 rad.

Structural abnormalities have been definitely observed at this level of radiation exposure. The period of time between 20 and 40 days following conception, therefore, appears to be more susceptible to this type of damage. Microcephaly is a more commonly induced defect in humans than other defects produced in lower animals. During the period of organogenesis, intrauterine doses of 25 rad or more may result in some retardation of growth which eventually might be recuperable. These types of changes have not been observed when the dose delivered was less than 10 rad. One should be reminded, as Table 2-1 indicates, that properly conducted diagnostic examinations including fluoroscopy of the abdomen (barium enema and upper GI's) should never deliver radiation of this magnitude and that the exposure should stay below the level of 2000 mrad.

No diagnostic examination involving ionizing radiation should be done without justification, and the expected benefit should outweigh the risk taken, no matter how small. The risk involved in such a properly conducted diagnostic procedure is very small indeed according to our scientific knowledge derived from experimental and epidemiological data including prospective and retrospective studies. (4) It is worth quoting here from NCRP's Report 54 that "no radiological examination for which there is a significant medical need should be denied to a patient, even if she is pregnant, for the risk to the patient of not having an indicated examination is also an indirect health risk to the embryo-fetus."

To this one could add that "the need for radiological examinations covers the entire spectrum of necessity, and health practitioners may, and often do, disagree on the importance of a given examination in a given situation." It goes without saying that the physician involved in the decision making for the examination of a pregnant woman should be familiar with the facts related to the amount of radiation involved per examination. The level below which no known harmful effects have been demonstrated (2000 mrad) should be taken into consideration, and the patient should be advised and a record should be kept of the patient's exposure.

DIAGNOSTIC ULTRASOUND DURING PREGNANCY: ANY RISK FACTORS INVOLVED?

It is pertinent in discussing diagnostic procedures during pregnancy to consider the biological implications and the significance of ultrasound, the most commonly performed imaging study of the pregnant woman. The use of ultrasonography and

the axiomatically accepted lack of any harmful biological effects
on the mother and fetus spectacularly increased the utilization
of this modality to the extent that it might sometimes be used
indiscriminately. The use of ultrasound in determing the gestational age, investigating the possibility of fetal abnormalities,
and following the fetal growth has become a routine and important clinical tool.

In addition, the use of ultrasound greatly facilitated making
important decisions for transfusion in utero and also evaluating
the need for intrauterine fetal therapy. The study of fetal vital
signs such as breathing, cardiac function, and movement have
become important in the field of research and for clinical studies. The use of real-time ultrasound imaging offered great
possibilities for the study of fetal physiology, which is also of
clinical importance.

Prior to the clinical application of ultrasound the examination
of the fetus was restricted to the auscultatory and physical examination. Application of radiography and fluoroscopy were
greatly restricted, particularly in view of the ionizing radiation
involved in this modality. The phenomenal increase in the utilization of ultrasound during pregnancy was encouraged, mainly
because of the lack of any known harmful effects of the ultrasound radiation. The overutilization, many times without clearly defined clinical indication, raises a serious question regarding the safety of the fetus exposed to the energy transmitted by
the ultrasound waves. In vitro ultrasound research studies as
well as observations on bacterial growth following exposure to
ultrasound waves indicated significant biological effects. (5) A
Food and Drug Administration study indicated the possible effects of ultrasound on the size and weight of the fetus. (1, 6, 17,
18)

Ultrasound also is the examination of choice, when applicable,
for pregnant women in conditions unrelated to pregnancy. Disease of the gallbladder, biliary tree and liver, and examination
of the kidneys, urinary bladder, and other abdominal organs
can be conducted without considering exposure to ionizing radiation.

An ultrasound beam is characterized by its frequency, its
duration, and the intensity of its beam. Of the three variables,
the one which probably has the most significant biological effect is the intensity and, of course, the time during which the
tissues are exposed to the ultrasound energy. It is known that
high intensities of ultrasound will result in an increase in the
temperature of the tissues exposed. (13, 14) It is also known
that increased temperatures have been proven to act as teratogens. (15) We should be quick to point out, however, that the

available ultrasound devices used in diagnosis operate at low intensities. Preliminary studies indicated the effects of ultrasound on cell cultures and particularly changes in DNA and also in cellular architecture and cellular motility including disturbances in the phagokinetic pattern.

The possibility that these changes might precipitate cellular activity eventually giving genesis to tumors has been postulated by Liebeskind. (16) It was also found that some of these changes in the cellular cultures persisted following exposure to ultrasound with findings of changes in subsequent generations of these exposed cells. (21) The clinical significance of these research findings remain unclear and have been questioned by other researchers. Undoubtedly further research in this direction will be of utmost importance. It is estimated that between 35 and 45% of all pregnant women in the United States are examined at least once with diagnostic ultrasound, and it is anticipated that with the current trend by the end of the 1980s every pregnant woman and her fetus will be exposed at least once to ultrasound diagnostic procedure. This impressive increase in the application of diagnostic ultrasound understandably raises the question of the possible risk to the mother and particularly to her fetus. Therefore, we should question the wisdom of the attitude of a significant number of physicians who consider the pregnancy itself to be an indication for a diagnostic ultrasound examination in order to reassure the pregnant woman and themselves that the pregnancy and the fetus are normal.

Against this background one always should consider the ultrasonic examination (as well as any other radiological examination and test) as a medical procedure from which the expected benefits outweigh the potential risks.

We should not consider a diagnostic ultrasonic examination only from the point of view of the "cost benefit ratio" but should also take into consideration the potential biological effects to the mother and the fetus. Our lack of more accurate information at the present time should make us cautious in the application of this most useful diagnostic modality. Of course no one will doubt the wisdom of using this test in high risk pregnancies or, for that matter, in any case where the physician anticipates useful information.

We believe that the knowledge of the possible adverse biological effects, particularly on the cell population of the fetus through the transfer of energy of ultrasound waves, should make the referring physician consider the indications for the examination. Once this concern is taken seriously I believe that any potential hazard will be well balanced by the indications. The ultrasonographer also should keep the time of exposure during the examination to the minimum necessary for the performance of an adequate study. It has been suggested that the record of all patients exposed to the ultrasound beam be kept in their files, including the length of the time of exposure and the energy factors used.

The energy transmitted by ultrasound produces heat in the internal structures including subcutaneous tissue, muscles, joints, and tendons. (13) According to Lehmann and Guy permanent elongation of tendons has been achieved following the therapeutic application of ultrasound by generating heat and with physical tension on the tendon. (14) Ultrasound has been used in physical therapy and in conjunction with stretching and motion exercises in order to improve limited joint motion. (14) Biological effects of ultrasound are not questioned. A direct quotation follows from a recent study by the U.S. Department of Health and Human Services (An Overview of Ultrasound: Theory, Measurement, Medical Applications and Biological Effects, 1982).

Benefits versus Risks: Choosing end points for study is especially difficult in human subjects. Latent periods easily could be as long as 20 years in the case of cancer development, or the effect may not be seen for another generation. The effects of ultrasound at diagnostic levels cannot necessarily be predicted from what we know to be the effects of therapeutic levels. Because the human fetus is sensitive to other forms of radiation there is considerable concern that it may also be sensitive to ultrasound. Thus, looking at prenatal exposure is a prudent step in investigating human effects. Until now, the fetus has been the focus of our concern; however, exposure of the mother could pose an equally or more significant risk. Animal studies suggest neurologic (sensory, cognitive, and developmental) immunologic and hematologic possibilities for study in humans. There is some evidence that if exposure is within the period of organogenesis, cogenital malformations may result from exposure to ultrasound in laboratory animals. In general, these end points in animal studies have been unexplored in humans and should be followed up wherever possible. Further, it must be realized that animal studies may not have explored all possible adverse effects, and it is quite possible that animal studies will not reveal some potential problems in humans.

It is obvious that with this basic background knowledge the physician taking care of any patient and particularly of a pregnant woman should always carefully examine the indications and the potential benefits of a diagnostic radiological examination. This includes not only the ones involving ionizing radiation but also any test with **potentially even minimal risks. This** primarily should determine the indications and the wisdom of the study. The cost effectiveness, although not the objective of this communication, also should be kept in mind when the potential benefits of the study are considered.

CONCLUSIONS

The recommendation for scheduling or postponing elective examinations with ionizing radiation, particularly when involving the abdomen or pelvis of women of childbearing capacity, should be guided by the following criteria:

1. If the examination of the abdomen is an elective one, meaning one that is not of immediate importance to the patient's health and therefore can be postponed to term should the patient prove to be pregnant, then postponement should be without any significant risk to the health of the patient or of her conceptus. Under these conditions the examination should not be done during pregnancy.

2. If the patient proves not to be pregnant, then the second consideration will be the timing of the examination. This should be related to the onset of the last menses. The examination should take place between 0 and 14 days from the onset of menses. The patient should be advised then to avoid pregnancy for two months. The examination should not be performed 15 days or more following the last menses. The advice to the patient is to postpone the examination until the next menstruation starts. If this does not occur and the patient proves to be pregnant, then this elective examination should be postponed until the termination of pregnancy.

3. If the physician is dealing with a known pregnant woman or if pregnancy cannot be ruled out and the examination is not an elective one, then the physician should advise the patient that the need for the examination outweighs the possible slight risk to the embryo or fetus. However, in this case the physician should consider and probably discuss with the radiologist the possibility of modifying the examination in

order to reduce to the dose to the uterus. If this can be done without any serious compromise to the examination, then the modified examination should be done. In case the examination cannot be modified without seriously compromising the examination, then the examination should proceed. This guideline should be carefully followed.

Concerning the use of ultrasound, as discussed in the text, no examination should be done without specific indication.

REFERENCES

1. Bierman, W. Ultrasound in the treatment of scars. Arch. Phys. Med. Rehabil., 209-214, 1954.

2. Brent, RL. Radiation teratogenesis. Teratology, 21:(3) 281-289, 1980.

3. Brent, RL, and Gorson, RO. Radiation exposure in pregnancy. Current Prob. Radiol., 11:1, 1972.

4. Bross, IDJ, and Natarajan, N. Risk of leukemia in susceptible children exposed to preconception, in utero and postnatal radiation. Preventative Med., 3:362, 1974.

5. Christoforidis, GA. The effects of airborne ultrasonic waves on the growth of bacillus, cereus and E. coli. Ohio J. Sci., 80:77, April 1980.

6. Stewart, HF, and Stratmeyer, ME. An overview of ultrasound: theory, measurement, medical applications and biological effects. Radiological Health, HHS Publication FDA 82-8190, July 1982.

7. Ford, DD, Patterson, JC, and Treuting, WL. Fetal exposure to diagnostic x-rays and leukemia and other malignant diseases in childhood. J. Nat'l Cancer Inst., 22:1093-1104, 1959.

8. Graham, S, Levin, ML, and Lilienfeld, AM. Methodological problems and design of the tristate leukemia survey. Ann. N.Y. Acad. Sci., 107:557-569, 1963.

9. Graham, S, Levin, ML, Lilienfeld, AM, et al. Preconception intrauterine and postnatal irradiation as related to leukemia. Nat'l Cancer Inst. Monogr., 19:347-371, 1966.

10. Holford, RM. The relation between juvenile cancer and obstetric radiography. Health Phys., 28:153, 1975.

11. Jablon, S, and Kato, H. Childhood cancer in relation to prenatal exposure to atomic bomb radiation. Lancet 2: 1000-1002, 1970.

12. Kato, H. Mortality of children exposed to the A-bomb while in utero, 1945-1969. Am. J. Epidemiology, 93:435-442, 1971.

13. Lehmann, JF, McMillan, JA, Bruner, GD, and Blumberg, JB. Comparative study of the efficiency of shortwave, microwave and ultrasonic diathermy in heating the hip joint. Arch. Phys. Med. Rehabil., 40:510-512, 1959.

14. Lehmann, JF, Masock, AJ, Warren, CG, and Koblanski, JN. Effects of therapeutic temperatures on tendon extensibility. Arch. Phys. Med., 51(8):481-487, 1970.

15. Lehmann, JF, and Guy, AW. Ultrasound therapy. In Interaction of Ultrasound and Biological Tissues. Reid, JM, and Sikov, MR, eds. HEW Publications FDA 73-8008, pp. 141-152, 1972.

16. Liebeskind, D, Bases, R, Elequin, F, Neubort, S, Leifer, R, Goldberg, R, and Koenigsberg, M. Diagnostic ultrasound: Effects on the DNA and growth patterns of animal cells. Radiology, 131(1):177-184, 1979.

17. Lyons, EA, Coggrave, M, and Brown, RE. Follow-up study in children exposed to ultrasound in utero — An analysis of height and weight in the first six years of life. In Proceedings of the 1980 Conference of the American Institute of Ultrasound in Medicine, p. 49, 1980.

18. Moore, RM, Barrick, MK, and Hamilton, PM. Effects of sonic radiation on growth and development. In Proceedings of the Society of Epidemiologic Research, p. 31, 1982.

19. Myrianthopoulos, NC. Preconception radiation, intrauterine diagnostic radiation, and childhood neoplasia. JNCI 65(4):681-685, 1980.

20. Neel, JV, Kato, H, and Schull, WJ. Mortality in the children of atomic bomb survivors and controls. Genetics, 76:311-325, 1974.

21. Pizzarello, DJ, Vivino, A, Madden, B, Wolsky, A, Keegan, AF, and Becker, M. Effect of pulsed low-power ultrasound on growing tissues. Exp. Cell Biol., 46(3): 179-191, 1978.

22. Pizzarello, DJ. Teratogenics effects of ionizing radiations and ultrasound. Prog. in Clin. Biol. Res., 44:67-76, 1980.

23. Stewart, A, and Kneale, GW. Radiation dose effects in relation to obstetric x-rays and childhood cancer. Lancet, 1:1185, 1970.

24. Stewart, A, Webb, J, and Hewitt, D. A survey of childhood malignancies. Brit. Med. J., 1:1495, 1958.

25. Totter, RJ, and McPherson, GH. Do childhood cancers result from prenatal x-rays? Health Phys., 40:(4)511-524, April 1981.

Chapter 3

TRAUMA IN PREGNANCY

Joe Sayre, M.D., and Neil R. Thomford, M.D.

Trauma is the fourth leading cause of death in the United States. It is the leading cause of death in people younger than 44 years old. At some time, 25% of all males and 10% of all females will be injured sufficiently to require a temporary absence from work. (1)

The peak incidence of trauma corresponds with childbearing years. Physicians caring for the injured, therefore, need to know the special physiologic changes related to pregnancy. They must also know how a gravid uterus may alter intra-abdominal arrangements and how this will alter both the physical exam and operative approach.

Minor accidents increase during pregnancy and are attributed to the protuberant abdomen and loosening of the pelvic joints. Serious accidents, however, do not show an increased frequency in pregnant women. (2)

Initial evaluation of the pregnant woman should be the same as for any accident victim. The "ABCs," urine output, and monitoring lines should be established as outlined in the Advance Trauma Life Support(3) and by numerous authors. The needs of the fetus can only be met if the needs of the mother are also met.

Predictable cardiovascular changes occur during pregnancy. A physiologic tachycardia of 15 to 20 beats/minute above base-line levels is present. Cardiac output is increased to 6 to 7 liters/minute even in the first trimester. (4) Peripheral vascular resistance is decreased and the systolic blood pressure is increased by 5 to 15 torr during the second trimester, but returns to normal at term. (1) Plasma volume is increased up to 50% above nonpregnant levels. (1, 4). Of this volume, up to 35% can be lost before symptoms of hypovolemia develop. (2) Uterine blood flow is sacrificed to preserve maternal blood flow by constriction of uterine arteries; adequate and rapid replacement of blood loss, therefore, is extremely important in pregnant patients. Vasoconstrictor drugs should be avoided because of marked sensitivity of the uterine arteries to these agents and the resulting limitation of blood flow to the uterus.

Central venous pressure (CVP) is not altered by pregnancy. (1) The CVP can and should be used as a guide to fluid replacement in young patients without cardiac or pulmonary disease. The use of a Swan-Ganz catheter is indicated in selected patients with dysfunction of multiple organ systems.

Electrocardiographic changes also occur during pregnancy. Elevation of the diaphragm by the enlarged uterus may cause left axis elevation of up to 15°. Supraventricular ectopy is a common occurrence. (1)

The respiratory rate is not altered in pregnancy but the tidal volume is increased by about 40%, with a corresponding decrease in residual volume. Arterial pCO_2 commonly falls to 30 mmHg by the third trimester. (1) These physiological changes must be considered when evaluating and managing the respiratory problems of the pregnant trauma victim. It is prudent to administer oxygen to the mother while the injuries are evaluated.

Positioning of the injured pregnant patient is very important. Inferior vena cava obstruction may be caused by the gravid uterus, resulting in a decrease in cardiac output. In addition, the elevated venous pressure in the lower half of the body may cause increased hemorrhage from injuries in that area. (2) The left-side-down position is preferred while awaiting diagnostic studies.

The administration of antibiotics is an established part of the management of nonpregnant patients with major injuries. When the injury victim is pregnant, the risk of the antibiotic to the fetus must be considered before deciding to administer the drug. Cephalosporins appear in amniotic fluid but are probably safe for the fetus. Aminoglycosides have been found to be concentrated in fetal kidneys. A significant number of newborns had hearing impairment after their mothers were treated with streptomycin for tuberculosis. Clindamycin rapidly crosses the placenta but little else about it is known. (5)

External fetal monitoring should be done while the patient is being evaluated. Fetal tachycardia is a sign of fetal distress in term infants. Loss of fetal beat-to-beat variability also suggests fetal distress. One must remember fetal heart rates may change without any change in maternal vital signs. (6)

Abdominal pericentesis is generally contraindicated in pregnancy. When it is performed, it should be done as an open procedure rather than via a percutaneously placed catheter.

The bladder should be emptied prior to the procedure. (3) Culdocentesis is an **acceptable alternative for determining intra-**abdominal bleeding. (3)

Amniocentesis may be used to determine potential fetal lung maturity and to determine if meconium is present in the amniotic fluid. The presence of meconium staining indicates that the fetus has undergone a period of acute anoxia. Immediate delivery should be considered if meconium is found, provided the fetal age is sufficient to suggest an excellent opportunity for survival. (2)

Pregnancy produces a variety of anatomical, physiological, and histological changes in the tissues and organs of the abdomen. The abdominal wall is stretched and its response to peritoneal irritation is reduced. (1) The intestines are displaced into the upper abdomen where they are partially protected by the rib cage. The risk of splenic rupture by blunt trauma does not appear to be increased during pregnancy. However, pregnancy may aggravate pre-existing splenic parenchymal disease or aneurysms. (1, 2, 7) Gastric motility is decreased and all patients should be assumed to have a full stomach. (1) The stomach of the pregnant patient with serious injuries should be emptied early during the course of their evaluation.

Because the uterus is protected by the bony pelvis in the first trimester, few ruptures have been reported before it projects from the pelvis. The bladder, bowels, and anterior abdominal wall cushion anterior blows, while the back muscles and the spine protect against posterior blows. The thickened uterine wall and the amniotic fluid help to protect the fetus during the second and third trimesters. (7) The uterus also protects the mother by dissipating the energy of impact. (2)

Penetrating abdominal injuries of pregnant patients should be managed according to the same principles as those applied to nonpregnant patients. Penetrating uterine wounds are rare and, in most instances, are gunshot wounds. (7) The uterus should be emptied if it limits effective exploration or if uterine bleeding cannot be controlled. Parametrial hemorrhage, common with penetrating wounds, demand careful evaluation and mature judgment since there are reports of uterine repair with subsequent vaginal delivery of normal infants.

Blunt uterine trauma is often associated with multiple organ injuries. Uterine rupture is rare but it can occur after apparently insignificant trauma. (7) The posterior wall of the fundus is the weakest point and is most susceptible to rupture. The site of placental attachment does not appear to influence the site of rupture. (2) The placenta is often injured with blunt abdominal trauma as it does not contain elastic tissue and cannot retract or expand. Uterine deformation with trauma may shear placental attachments but less than 10% of victims in severe collisions will have placental disruption. When it does occur, placental disruption may be recognized by blood in the vagina or by the presence of shock. In some instances, bleeding into the decidua may be self-limiting and not result in external bleeding. With significant placental disruption, the pregnancy will terminate spontaneously within 48 hours. If the fetus survives longer than 48 hours, harm from placental separation is unlikely. (2) Women with vaginal bleeding after trauma should be admitted to a hospital and observed for at least 48 hours.

Advanced placental separation may produce uterine tetany, shock, and disseminated intravascular coagulation. (2) Prompt uterine evacuation is needed. Necrosis of the chorionic endothelium liberates thromboplastin and activates the clotting mechanism. (9) Serial fibrogen and fibrin split-product laboratory values should be obtained, and fresh frozen plasma or cryoprecipitates used as needed to restore normal clotting function.

Amniotic fluid embolization may also occur. This is caused by sudden entry of the fluid through placental sinusoids or endocervical veins following uterine rupture, caesarean section, placenta previa, or abruptio placentae. The fluid may embolize to the kidneys, lungs, or brain and may be associated with hypofibrinogenemia. (9)

The decision to perform emergency caesarean section or hysterectomy is often difficult. Caesarean section is generally reserved for a patient with a viable, but compromised, fetus. When the fetus is known to be dead, sectioning may not be necessary. Hysterectomy is reserved for extensive uterine trauma with uncontrollable bleeding or inability to achieve adequate visualization when repairing extensive maternal intra-abdominal injuries. (2, 7, 8)

The use of seat belts should be continued during pregnancy since the greatest risk of injury in an auto accident occurs when the victim is thrown from the auto; seat belts keep the victim confined to the vehicle. Seat belts may be associated with a slight increase in fetal injury when accident victims wearing belts are compared to those not wearing belts and not thrown from the car, but this factor is not sufficient to ignore the added safety that accompanies wearing seat belts. (2, 10-12) The proper use of lap belts, placed over the pelvic bones, and shoulder straps is just as important and safe for the pregnant patient as for the nonpregnant patient.

REFERENCES

1. Buschbaum, H. (Ed.). Trauma in Pregnancy. Philadelphia, W. B. Saunders Co., 1977, pp. 1-38.

2. Crosby, WM. Trauma during pregnancy: Maternal and fetal injury. Obstet. Gynecol. Surv., 29(10):683, 1974.

3. Committee on Trauma. Advanced Trauma Life Support Course. American College of Surgeons, 1981.

4. Ueland, K. Maternal cardiovascular dynamics: VII, Intrapartum blood volume changes. Am. J. Obstet. Gynecol., 126(6):671, 1976.

5. Ledger, WJ. Antibiotics in pregnancy. Clin. Obstet. Gynecol. 20(2):411, 1977.

6. Katz, J, Hook, R, and Barash, P. Fetal heart rate monitoring in pregnant patients undergoing surgery. Am. J. Obstet. Gynecol., 125(2):267, 1976.

7. Dyer, I, and Barclay, DL. Accidental trauma complicating pregnancy and delivery. Am. J. Obstet. Gynecol., 83 (7):907, 1962.

8. Bochner, K. Traumatic perforation of the pregnant uterus. Obstet. Gynecol., 17(4):520, 1961.

9. Marx, G. Shock in obstetric patients. Anesthesiol., 26 (4):423, 1965.

10. Pepperell, RJ, Rubenstein, E, and MacIsacc, IA. Motor car accidents during pregnancy. Med. J. Aust., 1:203, 1977.

11. Lane, JC. Motor car accidents during pregnancy. 1 (letter). Med. J. Aust., 1:669, 1977.

12. Herbert, D, and Henderson, JM. Motor car accidents during pregnancy. 2 (letter). Med. J. Aust., 1:670, 1977.

Chapter 4

ENDOCRINE DISORDERS

Melissa Mash, M.D., George P. Grecos, M.D., and
Neil R. Thomford, M.D.

THYROID DISORDERS

Physiologic Changes During Pregnancy Related to the Thyroid Gland

The basal metabolic rate is increased during pregnancy on
the basis of extrathyroidal factors.(1) As a result pregnant
women frequently demonstrate signs and symptoms of hypermetabolism similar to those seen in hyperthyroidism. Tachycardia, palpitations, and heat intolerance are common. Increased vascularity and hyperplasia of the thyroid gland result
in a generalized enlargement of the thyroid in 50%-70% of normal pregnancies. This regresses after delivery. Production
of thyroxine-binding globulin (TBG) by the liver is increased as
a result of the elevated estrogen levels. As the thyroxine-
binding globulin level increases, the bound fraction of thyroxine
increases.

The total serum thyroxine (T_4) is the most frequently used
test of thyroid function. The protein-bound thyroxine and the bio-
logically active free thyroxine are measured by either radio-
immunoassay or competitive protein binding. In addition to being
elevated in over 95% of hyperthyroid patients, total T_4 is elevated
during pregnancy, in patients on estrogen therapy, and in patients with congenital elevation of thyroxine-binding globulin. In
the latter situations, however, the serum-free thyroxine concentration is normal. The free thyroxine level may be measured
but is usually estimated from the resin T_3 uptake. The total tri-
iodothyronine is also elevated in hyperthyroidism, pregnancy,
and other hypermetabolic states, and is measured by radioim-
munoassay. Free T_3 should be normal in pregnancy and can be
estimated by the resin T_3 uptake. (2-4)

Hyperthyroidism

Hyperthyroidism occurs in about 1 in 1500 pregnancies and is associated with an increase in frequency of premature labor and delivery, post-partum hemorrhage, and toxemia. (5) Graves' disease is responsible for 85% of the thyrotoxicosis in pregnancy. The remainder of the cases are caused by toxic nodular goiter, Hashimoto's thyroiditis, subacute thyroiditis, ficticious hyperthyroidism, iodine-induced hyperthyroidism, hyperemesis gravidarum, and hydatidiform mole. (6)

Hydatidiform moles occur in 1:2000 pregnancies and may cause hyperthyroidism or thyrotoxicosis because they produce a thyroid-stimulating factor. This factor is found to increase thyroid function in approximately 50% of the patients. The surgical removal of the mole is the treatment of choice although the patient may be treated medically with antithyroid medication until the operation.

The treatment of hyperthyroidism occurring during pregnancy depends upon the severity of the symptoms. (7) In mild cases specific therapy may not be increased. In severe cases medical or surgical treatment is required. Available agents for medical management include antithyroid drugs and adrenergic blocking agents. These agents cross the placenta and may affect the development of the fetus. The antithyroid drugs may suppress the thyroid function of the fetus and result in fetal goiter, hypothyroidism, and cretinism. The use of these drugs after delivery may be hazardous to the baby being breast fed since they are secreted in the mother's milk. Radioactive iodine is contraindicated by pregnancy.

Operation is indicated if medical therapy fails or prompt control is needed. Subtotal thyroidectomy may be performed with relative safety during pregnancy. (8) As with most operations during pregnancy it presents the least hazard to the fetus if done during the second trimester. (9)

Thyroid Nodules and Thyroid Cancer

Thyroid diseases commonly present as nodules of the thyroid gland. The incidence of thyroid nodules is greatest in females and increases with age. Thyroid nodules must first be differentiated from the physiologic enlargement of the thyroid gland often seen in pregnancy. (10) Every nodule must then be identified as benign or malignant: a history of radiation of the head or neck, (11,12) a family history of thyroid carcinoma, or a history of a rapidly growing painless nodule is suggestive of a thyroid malignancy. In the pregnancy age group a nodule which is solitary, hard, and is associated with cervical lymphadenopathy has a high probability of being malignant.

Aspiration and/or ultrasound examination will determine if the mass is solid or cystic. Needle biopsy may be needed for a definitive diagnosis. Fine needle aspiration is easy to perform in the office or on an out-patient basis with minimum risk. A 25-gauge needle is used and a smear is prepared. If carcinoma of the thyroid is found operation is needed.

Carcinoma of the thyroid gland is classified as papillary, follicular, medullary, and anaplastic carcinoma. It is common to have a mixed papillary and follicular carcinoma. These tumors may be considered as papillary carcinomas since their behavior is the same as the papillary carcinoma.

Papillary carcinoma is a slowly growing tumor which has a tendency to metastasize to the cervical lymph nodes. Even with metastases in cervical lymph nodes the survival is excellent. The treatment is surgical. A "near-total" thyroidectomy should be performed. When lymph nodes in the neck contain metastatic tumor a modified radical neck dissection should be done. For follicular carcinoma, a total thyroidectomy is recommended.

Medullary and anaplastic carcinoma are very rare during pregnancy. For medullary carcinoma a total thyroidectomy is recommended, although before any surgery, extensive workup to rule out the presence of other endocrine disorders should be performed. Medullary carcinoma may be familial and one component of the inherited multiple endocrine neoplasia type II syndrome.

Hypothyroidism During Pregnancy

Hypothyroidism is uncommon during pregnancy. Severe forms cause anovulation, infertility, and menometrorrhagia. Women with mild forms of hypothyroidism are able to conceive, but the incidence of spontaneous abortion, still birth, congenital abnormalities, and mental retardation of their children is high. Patients with subclinical hypothyroidism may become clinically hypothyroid because of the high metabolic demands during pregnancy. Women with hypothyroidism may become pregnant if treated adequately with hormonal supplements.

The treatment of a pregnant woman with hypothyroidism is essential. Since inadequate or inappropriate treatment continues to carry the risk of abortion, still birth, congenital abnormalities, and mental disorders of the fetus, the calculation of the appropriate dose of thyroxine is important in achieving euthyroidism. Thyroxine (0.1 to 0.2 mg daily) is usually sufficient to return the TSH, T_3, T_4, and TBI to normal range. The treatment should be started as early as possible because the incidence of abortion is highest during the first six weeks of pregnancy. Patients with clinical forms of hypothyroidism continue to be treated although they demand smaller amounts of thyroxine after delivery.

PARATHYROID DISORDERS

Normal Physiology — Physiologic Changes During Pregnancy

Calcium in serum exists in three different forms: ionized (60%), protein-bound mainly with albumin (35%), and salts with citrate, phosphate, and other ions (5%). The parathyroid hormone (PTH) regulates mainly the ionized calcium, the increase of which causes a decrease in the secretion of parathyroid hormone. During pregnancy calcium metabolism changes markedly. There is a significant amount of calcium transferred from mother to fetus (20-30 g daily), mostly in the last trimester. The relative hypocalcemia of the mother raises the secretion of the parathyroid hormone. Parathyroid hormone cannot cross the placenta but the calcium ion freely crosses the placenta and increases the serum calcium concentration in the fetus. This may cause suppression of the fetal parathyroid hormone secretions. After delivery, the parathyroid hormone hemostasis of mother and fetus returns to normal. (13, 14)

In a woman with hyperparathyroidism and high serum calcium level, excessive amounts of calcium cross the placenta and suppress the parathyroid hormone of the fetus. After the delivery the enormous calcium supply of the fetus suddenly diminishes, causing hypocalcemia and tetany.

Hyperparathyroidism

Hyperparathyroidism is very rare in pregnancy. The high parathyroid secretion and the elevated serum calcium levels are due to a solitary parathyroid adenoma in 80% to 85% of the cases. Multiple parathyroid adenomas, glandular hyperplasia, and carcinoma of the parathyroid gland comprise the remainder. Clinical manifestations of hyperparathyroidism include symptoms and findings involving the urinary system (calculi nephrocalcinosis, hematuria, polyuria), the gastrointestinal system (peptic ulcers, diarrhea, pancreatitis), the skeletal system (demineralization of bone, subperiosteal resorption, osteitis fibrosa cystica), the neuromuscular system (muscle weakness, fatigue, confusion, mental disorders), and symptoms from hypercalcemia such as anorexia, vomiting, constipation, dysphagia, and metallic taste. Often the patient is asymptomatic and the disease is recognized only after examination of the fetus identifies neonatal tetany, keratopathy, and bone deformities.

The critical laboratory finding is elevation of the serum calcium level although normocalcemic hyperparathyroidism has been reported. Serum phosphate is decreased and the urinary calcium is elevated. An elevated serum parathormone (PTH) level together with a high serum calcium confirms the diagnosis.

Differential diagnosis includes hypercalcemia in pregnancy, hyperthyroidism, hypervitaminosis D, milk alkali syndrome, parathormone-producing metastatic carcinoma, and sarcoidosis.

The definitive treatment is operation with excision of the adenoma or, when the pathology is parathyroid hyperplasia, removal of three and one-half glands.

Hypoparathyroidism

Hypoparathyroidism is not often seen during pregnancy. It is usually iatrogenic subsequent to operations on the thyroid and parathyroid glands. Since there is a physiologic reduction of the serum calcium level during pregnancy, subclinical forms which are not obvious before pregnancy become clinically significant during pregnancy. The most common symptom is tetany, which depends upon the serum concentration of ionized calcium, serum pH, total calcium concentration, and protein-binding calcium.

The differential diagnosis includes rickets, osteomalacia, steatorrhea, renal insufficiency with phosphorus retention, and hyperventilation. The treatment of the hypocalcemia during pregnancy requires a diet rich in calcium and low in phosphates, oral calcium administration (250 mg), and vitamin D (50,000 to 200,000 units per day). Patients who present with tetany may be treated by intravenous injection of calcium gluconate to relieve the symptoms.

Control of hypocalcemia in a pregnant woman is important since hypocalcemia may cause the baby to develop tetany, convulsions, or even heart block.

PITUITARY DISORDERS

Physiologic Changes During Pregnancy

During pregnancy the anterior pituitary gland enlarges to approximately twice the normal size, but changes do not occur in the posterior gland. The anterior gland gradually returns to normal size after pregnancy. All the cells of the anterior pituitary gland show increased activity resulting in an enormous production and release of hormones involved with the pregnancy process. A "pregnancy or transitional" cell can be identified which perhaps is specific to pregnancy and may be formed from the enlargement of a chromophobe or chromophil cell. In addition to the "pregnancy cell," both the eosinophil and basophil cells increase in number and size. (14)

Acromegaly

Acromegaly existing before pregnancy usually produces amenorrhea and infertility. Occasionally acromegaly may develop during pregnancy. Approximately 50 cases have been reported. Acromegaly is caused by acidophilic tumor cells which secrete excessive amounts of growth hormone and produce the characteristic facial and body appearance of acromegalic patients. Extension of the tumor outside the sella turcica may compress the optic chiasm and produce bitemporal hemianopsia. The clinical picture is complete with a number of other symptoms such as headaches, hypermetabolism, weight gain, and tongue enlargement. The treatment should not be delayed after pregnancy occurs. If the patient develops severe visual symptoms, hypophysectomy should be performed as soon as possible without anticipating any major effect on the pregnancy. Lactation, however, is usually inhibited. (15) Radiation treatment should be avoided during pregnancy because of the potentially hazardous effects on the fetus, but may be initiated after pregnancy.

Other Pituitary Adenomas

Chromophobe adenoma is the most common tumor of the pituitary. These tumors often produce headaches and visual symptoms. The tumor itself does not affect the pregnancy. However, if rapid growth comprises the patient's vision, hypophysectomy is indicated.

Basophilic adenomas produce increased secretion of ACTH and stimulate the adrenal cortex, which results in the development of Cushing's syndrome. The treatment of this tumor may be postponed until after pregnancy unless the rapid growth of the adenoma produces complications which demand prompt care. Hypophysectomy is the treatment of choice.

ADRENAL DISORDERS

Physiologic Changes During Pregnancy

The adrenal gland consists of the adrenal cortex and the medulla. The cortex has three layers. The outer zona glomerulosa secretes the mineral corticoids, the middle zona fasciculata secretes cortisol, and the inner zona reticularis secretes estrogen and androgen. Although the weight of the adrenal gland is not altered by pregnancy, the zona fasciculata is found to be markedly enlarged. (6,13,14)

During pregnancy, the serum aldosterone levels increase in response to sodium loss. Paralleling aldosterone secretion, renin levels also increase. This increase is minimal and does not cause hypertension in the pregnant woman.

The serum cortisol level starts increasing gradually at the end of the first trimester and reaches a level 2-4 times above normal. Most of the cortisol is bound to an alpha globulin, the transcortin, the production of which is controlled by the increasing production of estrogen. In addition to the increased cortisol production, a reduction of cortisol destruction contributes to the high cortisol levels. All adrenal hormone levels return to normal after delivery. (2)

The adrenal medulla secretes the catecholamines adrenaline and noradrenaline. These two hormones do not increase during pregnancy. There is a transient increase in both hormones during labor, but levels return to normal within 20 minutes after delivery. This increase is attributable to the stress of delivery.

Cushing's Syndrome

Extensive production of glucocorticoid hormones can be caused by adrenocortical hyperfunction secondary to diffuse hyperplasia, adenoma, or carcinoma of the adrenal cortex. Diffuse hyperplasia is the result of extensive secretion of ACTH from a pituitary adenoma. Chronic administration of corticosteroids can also cause the syndrome. (2)

The clinical complex consists of the characteristic truncal obesity, hypertension, hirsutism, amenorrhea, striae, poor wound healing, thin skin, "easy" bruising, weakness, acne, and mental disorders. Since amenorrhea and infertility are common features of Cushing's syndrome, pregnancy is rare. Fewer than 30 cases of Cushing's syndrome and pregnancy have been reported.

Treatment should start as early as possible before complications develop. If the cause is located in the adrenals, bilateral or unilateral adrenalectomy should be done. In pituitary-dependent disease, the treatment should be directed to the pituitary. Transsphenoidal hypophysectomy is a relatively safe procedure. Radiation therapy may be hazardous during pregnancy but is recommended after delivery. Bilateral adrenalectomy for pituitary-dependent disease should be avoided during pregnancy. The patients should have an appropriate steroids supplement during and after surgery.

Primary Aldosteronism (Conn's Syndrome)

Primary aldosteronism is very rare in pregnancy. This syndrome is caused in most instances by an aldosterone-secreting adenoma of the adrenal cortex. The presentation of the disease is characterized by hypertension, hypokalemia, muscle weakness, and metabolic alkalosis. The serum aldosterone level is elevated, and renin production by the kidney is suppressed. (2)

Diagnosis is difficult because the syndrome is very rare and the symptoms are similar to those of normal pregnancy. The findings of a high serum aldosterone level and a low renin level are important in making the diagnosis. An intravenous pyelogram, tomograms, and computerized tomography all may be helpful tests but the decision to obtain one or more of these examinations must depend on a careful assessment of the potential risks and benefits.

Surgical removal of the adenoma is the treatment of choice. Occasionally, treatment with spirolactone can temporarily suppress the adenoma and control the syndrome until operation.

Adrenal Cortical Insufficiency

Women with adrenal cortical insufficiency may maintain menstruation or may have amenorrhea, but conception is rare in untreated patients. (2) With hormonal replacement therapy, more women with adrenal cortical insufficiency have become pregnant.

Primary destruction of the adrenal by disease, surgery, or inadequate secretion of ACTH from the pituitary may cause the syndrome. The signs and symptoms are nausea, vomiting, weight loss, weakness, fatigue, increased pigmentation, hypotension, hypoglycemia, vertigo, and syncopy. Stress is usually the trigger for the presentation of the syndrome.

Treatment consists of gluco- and mineralocorticoid replacement. Hydrocortisone (20-30 mg daily) or cortisone acetate (37.5 mg daily) are usually enough to satisfy the daily metabolic requirements. Adequate amounts of salt must be included in the diet. Delivery, by either natural means or caesarean section, is considered equivalent to a major operation. Hydrocortisone (100 mg) is given before delivery, followed by 100 mg every 6 hours during the next 24 hours. The return to normal replacement dosage should be accomplished through a gradual decrease over the following 8-10 days.

Infants born to mothers with adrenal cortical insufficiency who received extensive doses of corticosteroids, have a lower birth weight than those of the same gestational age and may have impairment of the adrenal function at birth.

Pheochromocytoma

Pheochromocytomas are tumors causing hypersecretion of catecholamines. They are found in 0.1% to 0.5% of the general population and approximately 2% of hypertensive patients. Pheochromocytoma can exist as an isolated disease, or as part of a multiple endocrine adenopathy (MEA II and IIb) coexisting with thyroid medullary carcinoma, hyperparathyroidism, and submucosal neuromas. (1)

Pheochromocytoma during pregnancy is dangerous, with a mortality rate of 40%-50%. Most deaths occur at or immediately after delivery. The fetal mortality rate is approximately 55%. A lower mortality rate (15%-20%) occurs in cases in which the diagnosis is made before the end of pregnancy. A less favorable prognosis exists for cases in which the diagnosis is made during delivery (58%).

Clinical manifestations of pheochromocytoma include hypertension (90%), presenting as sustained hypertension or paroxysmal attacks, headaches (80%), palpations, pallor, nausea, tremor, dyspnea, blurring vision, excessive perspiration, and fainting. The patient may have only mild hypertension or may have the entire spectrum of symptoms.

Diagnosis is made from the excessive catecholamine level in plasma and urine. Vanillylmandelic acid (VMA) is elevated in 90% of the patients, but false positive results may be caused by drugs or diet. Measurement of urinary metanephrine excretion is most accurate because it is unaffected by diet and drugs. Provocative tests such as histamine or phentolamine should be avoided because they may provoke hypertensive crisis. Abdominal x-ray, computerized tomography, intravenous pyelogram, tomograms of the kidneys, and arteriography all carry risks but should be performed if necessary.

The treatment of choice is the surgical removal of the tumor. Alpha blocking agents and occasionally beta blockers can be used to control the high blood pressure. Alpha blockers such as phentolamine control the blood pressure during surgery, and beta blockers such as propranolol effectively control the tachycardias.

During the first two trimesters of pregnancy a midline abdominal incision for bilateral adrenal tumors provides an excellent approach. When the tumor is unilateral, a flank incision is preferred. For diagnoses made in the third trimester, when fetal maturity is well developed, the abdominal approach is recommended. Delivery by caesarean section and tumor removal should be performed simultaneously. In high risk cases, most authors advocate removal of the tumor regardless of the stage of pregnancy and the risk to the fetus.

REFERENCES

1. Pritchard, JA, and Macdonald, PC. William's Obstetrics, 16th ed. New York, Appleton-Century-Crofts, 1980, pp. 249-253, 748-751.

2. Montgomery, DAD, and Harley, JMG. Endocrine disorders. Clin. Obstet. Gynecol. , 4:339-371, 1977.

3. Osathanondh, R. Endocrine tests in obstetrics and gynecology — Part I. In Current Problems in Obstetrics and Gynecology. Chicago, Year Book Medical Publishers, 1980.

4. Osathanondh, R, and Lackritz, RM. Endocrine tests in obstetrics and gynecology — Part II. In Current Problems in Obstetrics and Gynecology. Chicago, Year Book Medical Publishers, 1980.

5. Burrow, GN. Hyperthyroidism during pregnancy. New Engl. J. Med. , 298:150-153, 1978.

6. Romney, SL, Gray, MJ, and Little, AB. Diseases complicating pregnancy. Gynecol. Obstet. , 2:753-760, 1981.

7. Ben Zion, T. Manual of Gynecologic and Obstetric Emergencies. Philadelphia, W. B. Saunders, 1979.

8. Mestman, JH. Management of thyroid diseases in pregnancy. Clin. Perinatol. , 7:371-385, 1980.

9. Gottesman, RL, and Refetoff, S. Diagnosis and management of thyroid diseases in pregnancy. J. Reprod. Med. , 11:19-22, 1973.

10. Burrow, GN. Thyroid and parathyroid function in pregnancy. Endocrinol. Preg. , 2:246-270, 1977.

11. Asteris, GT, and DeGroot, LJ. Thyroid cancer: Relationship to radiation exposure and to pregnancy. J. Reprod. Med. , 17:209-216, 1976.

12. Block, MA. Surgery of thyroid nodules and malignancy. Current Problems in Surgery, Chicago, Year Book Medical Publishers, 1983.

13. Salem, R, and Taylor, S. Hyperthyroidism in pregnancy. Br. J. Surg, 66:648-650, 1979.

14. Wilson, JR, and Carrington, ER. Medical and surgical complications during pregnancy. Obstet. Gynecol. , 38:816-820, 1979.

15. Kelly, WF, Doyle, FH, Mashiter, K, et al. Pregnancies in women with hyperprolactinaemia: Clinical course and obstetric complications of 41 pregnancies in 27 women. Br. J. Obstet. Gynecol. , 86:698-705, 1979.

Chapter 5

GASTROINTESTINAL DISEASES DURING PREGNANCY

George P. Grecos, M.D., and Neil R. Thomford, M.D.

Surgical problems of the GI tract are the most frequently encountered nonobstetric complications seen during pregnancy (Table 5-1). (1) Of all pregnancies, more than two-thirds are completed uneventfully. Of the remaining one-third, one-half are terminated in an abortion and the other half are complicated by a variety of disorders which threaten the mother, the fetus, or both. Gastrointestinal problems requiring operation occur in 0.5% of all pregnancies. (2) The prompt diagnosis of these problems is difficult because some of the signs and symptoms of "normal" pregnancy are similar to those of acute abdominal disease. The morbidity of GI complications is magnified by any delay in diagnosis and/or treatment. This is particularly true when the complication is an abdominal illness.

When evaluating the pregnant patient for a possible abdominal disorder the anatomical and functional changes associated with pregnancy must be considered. Anatomical changes include displacement of intraperitoneal organs, such as the appendix, thereby increasing the difficulty of making a diagnosis of appendicitis. An example of the functional changes is the increase in intra-abdominal pressure with compression of the inferior vena cava and iliac veins, causing varicose veins and hemorrhoids.

Physiological Changes of the GI Tract During Pregnancy

During pregnancy, the appetite increases and the threshold of taste heightens. The enzymatic activity of saliva decreases and smooth muscles of the uterus, bowel, ureters, and blood vessels have less tone. Contractions of the esophagus are increased in magnitude while the lower esophageal sphincter pressure is decreased. Secretion of gastric acid is reduced

Table 5-1   Surgical Problems of the GI System During
           Pregnancy

Problem	Percent
Appendicitis	60
Trauma	15
Biliary tract	10
Bowel obstruction	4
Anorectal	3
Tumors	2
Peptic ulcers	2
Inflammatory disease of small and large bowels	1.5
Miscellaneous	0.5

and the motility of the stomach, small bowel, and large bowel
is decreased. Secretion of amylase and lipase by the pancreas
is diminished. During the early stages of pregnancy, the patient
may develop nausea and vomiting, leukocytosis, abnormal liver
function, constipation, increased blood pressure, etc. (3,4)
These symptoms and findings may be only those associated
with a normal pregnancy, or they may be caused by gastrointestinal disease. Close observation and continuous monitoring
and evaluation of the patient is mandatory for prompt diagnosis
and treatment. The need for operation during pregnancy may
be the result of the exacerbation of pre-existing disease or the
development of a new problem. Finally, the illness causing
the patient's symptoms may or may not be related to the current pregnancy. An awareness of these general considerations
is essential when evaluating pregnant patients with symptoms
and signs suggestive of abdominal disease.

ACUTE ABDOMEN DURING PREGNANCY

The etiology of an "acute abdomen" is the same in the pregnant as in the nonpregnant patient. The recognition of acute ab-

dominal disease in the pregnant patient is, however, more difficult since the symptoms which suggest acute abdominal problems (pain, nausea, vomiting, and distention of the abdomen) often accompany a normal pregnancy. (5) A thorough knowledge of the symptoms and signs of normal pregnancy will allow proper interpretation of these findings. (6) Nausea and vomiting are common in early pregnancy; their occurrence after the fourth month should suggest an etiology other than pregnancy. Abdominal distention caused by pregnancy should have a symmetrical appearance. Asymmetrical distention may be the result of abnormal intra-abdominal processes such as an ovarian cyst or a uterine fibroid. Rapid distention combined with other symptoms, may indicate the presence of mechanical bowel obstruction or a dynamic ileus from peritonitis. The problem of diagnosis of acute abdominal disease during pregnancy is further compounded by the increase in the blood volume, the leukocyte count, the erythrocyte sedimentation, and the decrease in blood hemoglobin and hematocrit associated with pregnancy. The uninformed physician may be misled by laboratory findings reflectting these changes and misinterpret them as signs of disease.

The management of acute abdominal disease, be it medical or surgical, will of course be based on the general condition of the patient, the probable or established diagnosis, the usual considerations including the time interval from the onset of symptoms, and the stage of pregnancy. The progress of acute abdominal disease is accelerated during pregnancy due to the increase in blood flow in the intraperitoneal tissues and organs. Therefore, for those problems which require operation, an early decision and prompt operation are essential. (7) When the diagnosis and need for operation are in doubt, frequent repeated evaluations are mandatory to avoid delays in operation. In general, it is necessary to consider operation for the pregnant patient for fewer findings and findings of less magnitude than required for the nonpregnant patient.

Gastrointestinal Bleeding During Pregnancy

Gastrointestinal bleeding is less frequent and less severe in pregnant patients than in comparable groups of nonpregnant patients. (8) Massive bleeding is extremely rare. (9,10) The causes of bleeding during pregnancy are similar to those of the nonpregnant patient (Table 5-2).

It is well known that gastric ulcer disease is less common in women than in men. (11) In a pregnant woman, the incidence of gastric ulcer disease is even less frequent and is easy to control because of the diminished gastric acid secretion and the reduced gastric motility. Aspirin and other analgesics often

Table 5-2   Causes of Bleeding During Pregnancy

1. Gastric ulcer	9. Granulomatous colitis
2. Salicylates	10. Angiomas
3. Steroids	11. Diverticulitis
4. Mallory-Weiss syndrome	12. Small bowel diseases
5. Hiatal hernia with reflux esophagitis	13. Tumors or Meckel's diverticulum
6. Esophageal varices	14. Parasites
7. Hemorrhagic gastritis	15. Hemorrhoids (other than cancer)
8. Ulcerative colitis	

used by pregnant women for mild discomfort or pain are probably the most common cause of upper GI bleeding. Erosive esophagitis with or without hiatal hernia is a relatively common cause of upper GI bleeding during pregnancy. Hyperemesis gravidarum may complicate pregnancy and may result in upper GI bleeding either from Mallory-Weiss syndrome or erosive esophagitis. Pregnant women on treatment with steroids for hyperemesis gravidarum or another illness may develop hemorrhagic gastritis or even gastric perforation.

Small bowel disorders which may cause gastrointestinal bleeding during pregnancy include hemangiomas, parasitic diseases, neoplasms, and ectopic gastric mucosa in a Meckel's diverticulum. The common finding in these cases is blood mixed with the stool which varies in color from black to bright red, depending upon the severity of the bleeding.

Ulcerative or granulomatous colitis is an extremely unusual cause of bleeding during pregnancy but bloody diarrhea must suggest the possibility of colitis. These patients deserve special attention because toxic megacolon is a potential complication which may be fatal for the mother and the fetus. Other potential sources of bleeding from the colon are hemangiomas, other neoplasms, diverticulosis, and parasitic diseases. Compression of the pelvic veins by the gravid uterus, combined with constipation which is common during pregnancy, causes stasis in the hemorrhoidal veins. The passage of small amounts of bright red blood before or after defecation is not unusual. Massive bleeding from hemorrhoids is rare.

Diagnosis

The symptoms and signs of GI bleeding in the pregnant patient are the same as for the nonpregnant patient. The past medical history and a detailed description of the present illness are essential to suggest the diagnosis. Aspiration of the stomach should be done routinely in an attempt to document the proximal GI tract as the site of hemorrhage; the absence of blood in the gastric aspirate does not rule out bleeding from the duodenum. Appropriate endoscopic examinations may identify the source. Finally, radiologic examinations including barium contrast studies and arteriography may be needed but each must be selected and utilized after careful weighing of the benefits and risks to both the mother and fetus.

Treatment

Since the fetus is threatened by hypovolemia and/or anemia, prompt intravenous infusion of fluids and blood, when appropriate, is essential. Lavage of the stomach with a cold saline solution and the instillation of antacids will stop bleeding from the stomach and duodenum in most cases. (11) Cimetidine and similar drugs are not recommended until bleeding has been arrested since there is evidence to suggest they increase mucosal blood flow. Recurrence may be prevented in most instances by maintaining the pH of the gastric aspirate at or above 5 with H_2 antagonists and antacids. If medical management fails, exploratory laparotomy with control of bleeding is necessary. Embolization of the bleeding vessel through an angiographic catheter may be indicated in selected patients. Balloon tubes and sclerotherapy may be needed if the hemorrhage is from gastroesophageal varices. The use of vasopressin is, of course, contraindicated in the pregnant patient. In some patients in the last trimester of pregnancy, delivery of the fetus by caesarean section may be indicated at the time of operation to control gastrointestinal hemorrhage.

Peptic Ulcer Perforation

Perforation of a peptic ulcer is an extremely rare occurrence during pregnancy. Becker-Anderson et al. were able to collect only 31 documented cases. (12) In their review, perforation

usually occurred in the third trimester or in the immediate
postpartum period. The presenting symptom is most often sudden, severe epigastric pain. Epigastric or diffuse tenderness
is common with the "board-like" abdomen being pathognomonic
of gastric acid in the peritoneal cavity. Identification of "free"
intraperitoneal air with plain upright or lateral decubitus roentgenograms of the abdomen is possible in only 60% to 65% of
cases. The potential risks and benefits must be weighed when
considering the ordering of this diagnostic study. When a diagnosis of perforated ulcer is made, operation is mandatory and
should be performed expediently. Closure of the perforation is
the operation of choice.

Acute Appendicitis

Acute appendicitis is the most common gastrointestinal
problem requiring an operation during pregnancy. The incidence
of acute appendicitis during pregnancy varies from 1 in every
700 to 1 in every 2700. When a series of more than 500,000 deliveries was reviewed, the overall incidence was 1 in 1500.

Age

Acute appendicitis during pregnancy has its highest incidence
between age 20 and 25 years. The multiparous woman appears
to be at greater risk, with the incidence of acute appendicitis
being directly proportional to the number of pregnancies. (13,14)

Symptoms

Abdominal pain is the predominant symptom. Like the pain
of appendicitis in the nonpregnant patient, it commonly begins
in the periumbilical region and "shifts" to the right lower quadrant of the abdomen. In the last trimester of pregnancy, the
pain, when "localized" to the right abdomen, may be in the
right flank rather than the right lower quadrant due to the displacement of the appendix by the enlarged uterus. (15,16) Nausea
and/or vomiting are the next most common symptoms and are
most frequent in the second and third trimester. (15) When the
patient is in the first trimester of pregnancy, the clinician must
be careful not to confuse the nausea and vomiting of appendicitis
with that which occurs with an uncomplicated pregnancy. Anorexia is present in more than 50% of cases of appendicitis.
Fever and tachycardia are findings in approximately 20% of patients. The abdominal findings are similar to those of the nonpregnant woman. Right lower quadrant tenderness with or without

rebound tenderness is the most common and important finding. Digital examination of the rectum may identify tenderness in the right pelvis but is not as reliable a sign as it is in nonpregnant patients. (17)

Laboratory examinations are valuable in excluding urinary tract infections and other diseases which may be confused with appendicitis. No test is diagnostic of appendicitis; even the value of the leukocyte count is diminished by the usual leukocytosis of pregnancy — 8000 to 12,000 per cubic millimeter.

The likelihood of abortion or premature labor after operation is slight unless perforation of the appendix and peritonitis have occurred. In the series reported by the senior author (NRT), the single abortion which followed appendectomy occurred in one of two patients who had a perforated appendix. Abortion in one of the seven patients in whom the diagnosis of appendicitis was in error was caused by peritonitis secondary to perforation of a fallopian tube abscess.

When a diagnosis of acute appendicitis is made, operation should be performed promptly. (18) The mortality of appendicitis during pregnancy is often referred to as the mortality of "delay," as reported by Barber and Graber. (2) Preoperative preparation is an individual problem but one must be concerned with precautions to avoid hypotension or hypoxia during or after the operation. (19,20) Appropriate antibiotics should be given prior to operation. The value of administering progesterone before and after the operation is uncertain. However, progestational agents may be of aid in preventing premature labor or abortion. The authors administer progesterone to all patients undergoing an operation during pregnancy unless the patient is at term.

A muscle-splitting incision is preferable. It may be desirable to make the incision more cephalad than usual when the patient is in the third trimester of pregnancy. Caesarean section has been successfully combined with appendectomy by Meiling, but recent publications favor appendectomy alone in instances of acute appendicitis during labor or when the patient is near term. When perforation of the appendix has occurred, intraoperative management is determined by the extent of the peritonitis. A localized collection of pus may be removed with sponges, while widespread peritonitis may require lavage of the abdomen and the placement of intraperitoneal drains brought through individual small wounds in the abdominal wall. If the diagnosis is in error, the abdominal cavity must be searched for other evidence of disease of other organs. This may require enlargement of the initial incision. (22)

Maternal and Fetal Mortality

Though both maternal and fetal mortality of appendicitis has dramatically decreased in recent years, it still remains high. Maternal mortality increases with the duration of the pregnancy. In 1960, Black reported no maternal mortality in the first trimester, 3. 9% in the second, 10. 9% in the third, and 16. 7% in the intrapartum period. In 1967, Brant reported no maternal deaths in the first two trimesters but a 7. 3% mortality in the third trimester.

The fetal mortality has decreased from 34%-40% in 1950 to 8. 7% today. In cases of peritonitis, the fetal mortality rate remains high, but in nonperforated appendicitis it is only 1. 5%. The most important factor in reducing mortality is early diagnosis and operation while the infection is still localized.

Bowel Obstruction

The incidence of mechanical bowel obstruction during pregnancy ranges from 1 in 3600 to 1 in 66,430 deliveries. The most common cause of bowel obstruction during pregnancy is adhesions resulting from abdominal operations. In contrast to the nonpregnant population, femoral and inguinal hernias account for less than 5% of intestinal obstructions. This may be the result of the enlarged uterus displacing the bowel from the pelvis. Neoplasms also are an uncommon cause of obstruction. (21)

The most common site of obstruction is the small bowel. (23) When obstruction of the colon occurs it is usually due to sigmoid volvulus. A unique cause of large bowel obstruction in pregnancy and sometimes in the early postpartum period is the compression of the sigmoid colon against the pelvic rim by an enlarged uterus.

Mechanical bowel obstruction associated with pregnancy occurs most often at:

1. The fifth month (16-18 weeks) when the uterus becomes an intraperitoneal organ and stretches adhesions in the pelvis and lower abdomen.

2. When the head is "engaged" in the pelvis (9th month, 36-38 weeks).

3. Immediately after delivery when the size of the uterus is suddenly reduced.

The symptoms are the same as for the nongravid patient: diffuse colicky pain, nausea and vomiting, and abdominal distention. When obstruction occurs in the third trimester, the symptoms may be erroneously attributed to the onset of labor. Cramping abdominal pain and high-pitched bowel sounds, as in the nonpregnant patient, should suggest mechanical obstruction. The degree of abdominal distention will vary with the level of obstruction. When the obstruction is in the proximal small intestine vomiting occurs early, cramping pain is not a consistent symptom, and distention is uncommon. With obstruction of the large intestine distention occurs early and vomiting late if at all. Vomiting may result in dehydration and the characteristic hypokalemic hypochloremic alkalosis.

Endoscopy may confirm obstructions of the colon but roentgenograms of the abdomen, despite their potential risk early in pregnancy, may be needed to identify mechanical obstruction of the small intestine.

Management

Correction of fluid and electrolyte imbalance is the initial goal since any hypotension or hypoxia will threaten both the fetus and the mother. A nasogastric should be inserted to decompress the stomach. If mechanical obstruction is confirmed an exploratory laparotomy should be performed without delay. An exception is the patient with sigmoid volvulus. Before advising operation, one should attempt relief by endoscopy and the insertion of a rectal tube.

Acute Pancreatitis

The incidence of acute pancreatitis during pregnancy ranges from 1 in 1000 to 1 in 10,000. The etiology is similar to that in the nonpregnant woman. Chololithiasis is the most common cause, and alcohol abuse ranks second. (24) Additional causes include hyperlipidemia, steroid therapy, trauma, hypothyroidism, vasculitis, and a variety of medications. Pancreatitis can occur during any stage of pregnancy, however, more than half of the cases occur in the last trimester. Two possible reasons are (1) the physiologic hyperlipidemia which appears in the third trimester of pregnancy and (2) the treatment of third trimester edema with chlorothiazides. Both chlorothiazides and hyperlipidemia are established predisposing factors for women. Acute, severe, steady epigastric pain radiating to the back is the characteristic symptom. Nausea, vomiting, bloating, and

jaundice may also be present. On clinical examination there is
often epigastric tenderness, abdominal distention, and hypo-
active bowel sounds. Fever, tachycardia, and hypovolemic
shock may indicate hemorrhagic pancreatitis.

Elevation of serum and/or urinary amylase content provides
the best laboratory evidence of pancreatitis but the degree of
rise does not correlate with the severity of the disease. Other
laboratory findings include hypoglycemia, glycosuria, leukocytosis, increased serum and urine bilirubin, and decreased
serum calcium and serum albumin. The plain abdominal x-rays
may disclose gallstones, an isolated "sentinel" loop of distended
small intestine, or fluid in the left pleura space.

The prognosis is poor when the patient has a leukocyte count
above 16,000/ml, a blood glucose concentration over 200 ml%,
a blood urea nitrogen more than 5 ml%, a serum calcium level
below 6 mg/100 ml, and arterial PO_2 below 60 mmHg, or an
estimated fluid sequestration of more than 6000/ml.

Treatment

The treatment of acute pancreatitis during pregnancy is the
same as in nonpregnant women. Nasogastric suction and restriction of oral intake are necessary. Fluid and electrolyte
replacement for this "internal burn" should insure a urine output of more than 30 ml/hour. When there is a severe pancreatitis with marked loss and/or sequestration of fluid the placement of a central venous catheter or Swan-Ganz catheter may
be indicated. For analgesia, Demerol (meperidine) is recommended. In severe cases the administration of intravenous
cimetidine may prevent hemorrhagic gastritis.

Most cases of pancreatitis subside with medical management.
Surgical treatment is necessary only in the following circumstances: (1) if exploration of the abdomen is necessary because
the diagnosis is uncertain, (2) to correct disease of the biliary
system in instances where the patient is not responding to medical treatment, and (3) to treat complications such as pancreatic abscess, necrosis, pseudocyst, and pancreatic ascitis.

The mortality for pancreatitis during pregnancy has been
reported to be as high as 21%. (56) In an editorial, H. R. Barber and E. A. Graber suggest that caesarean section for patients in the late stages of pregnancy may be indicated since
dramatic recovery has been reported after delivery of the baby.
However, Benson (1) has commented that pregnancy does not
alter the course of pancreatitis and that pregnancy is not influenced by this disorder.

Nausea and Vomiting of Pregnancy and
Its Associated Complications

During early pregnancy, the incidence of nausea and vomiting is reported to be between 25% and 40%. The etiology is uncertain, however, hormonal, environmental, and psychosomatic factors may all have an etiologic role. (25) A small number of patients (approximately 3 or 4 per 1000 deliveries) develop intractable vomiting known as "hyperemesis gravidarum." Hypovolemia and electrolyte imbalance are potential sequelae. Complications of this condition which may require emergency surgical intervention include mucosal tears at the gastroesophageal junction (Mallory-Weiss syndrome) and rupture of the distal thoracic esophagus (Boerhaave's syndrome). The Mallory-Weiss syndrome presents as an acute upper GI bleed. Medical management is usually sufficient but occasionally persistent hemorrhage may require exploratory laparotomy and suturing of the gastric mucosal tears.

Boerhaave's syndrome commonly presents with acute excruciating pain in the epigastrium and left lower thorax. An ipsilateral pleura effusion is a common finding, and roentgenograms of the chest may identify air in the mediastinum. The diagnosis can be confirmed by fluoroscopy after instilling water-soluble contrast in the esophagus or by endoscopy with direct visualization of the perforation. The prognosis is better if the esophagus is repaired within 12 hours of the rupture. When the interval between rupture and operation is greater than 12 hours more radical procedures may be necessary.

Esophageal Hiatus Hernia and Dysfunction of the
Lower Esophageal Sphincter

Swallowing is based upon the normal function of (1) the muscles of the pharynx and the upper esophageal sphincter, (2) the smooth muscle of the esophagus, and (3) the lower esophageal sphincter. Although there is a significant pressure difference between the thoracic and the abdominal cavities, the stomach remains in the abdomen because of the anatomy of the esophageal hiatus and the gastroesophageal ligament. (26) A competent lower esophageal sphincter prevents regurgitation of gastric contents into the esophagus. When an anatomic derangement of this area exists, the higher intra-abdominal pressure "pushes" a portion of the stomach through the esophageal hiatus of the diaphragm resulting in a "hiatus hernia."

There are two types of hiatus hernia. A sliding hiatus hernia is one in which gastroesophageal junction moves up through the hiatus into the thorax. A paraesophageal hernia is so named because the gastroesophageal junction remains in normal position while the herniated part of the stomach passes through the hiatus alongside the esophagus. In the first type, the lower esophageal sphincter is usually incompetent and there is reflux of contents into the esophagus. In the second type, the lower esophageal sphincter remains intact and there is no regurgitation.

During pregnancy, hormonal factors decrease the tone of the gastroesophageal sphincter. This, together with the increased intra-abdominal pressure (especially in the last trimester), results in regurgitation of gastric contents. Regurgitation of gastric juice damages the esophageal squamous epithelium, producing esophagitis. When severe and prolonged, the regurgitation may cause an esophageal stricture. Occasionally an incompetent pyloric sphincter exists with a sliding hiatus hernia. In this case the alkaline content of the duodenum may regurgitate back through the stomach into the esophagus and produce alkaline esophagitis.

The incidence of hiatal hernia is directly related to the number of pregnancies. With one pregnancy the incidence is 5%, but for multiparous women it is 18-20%. After delivery the majority of hernias are no longer demonstrable. A presumptive diagnosis of hiatus hernia may be made by clinical examination. If the severity of the patient's symptoms and/or lack of response to medical treatment justify additional studies then an upper gastrointestinal series or endoscopy may be indicated, with the choice being dependent on several factors including the stage of the pregnancy.

Treatment

Both hiatus hernia and heartburn occur in late pregnancy. The usual time of appearance is the middle of the second trimester. To prevent reflux esophagitis the patient should use several pillows when sleeping and avoid laying down immediately after eating. She should be instructed to eat frequent small meals and refrain from coffee, carbonated beverages, and smoking. Antacids are also helpful. Operation is rarely necessary during pregnancy. When needed, the Nissen fundoplication is the procedure of choice.

Gallbladder Disorders

The development of gallstones is commonly associated with pregnancy. Etiologic factors include the delay in emptying of the gallbladder during pregnancy (especially in the third trimester), displacement and kinking of the extrahepatic biliary tree from the enlarged uterus, and biliary stasis with an increased cholesterol concentration in bile. (27) The diagnosis of gallstones is frequently made in the first postpartum year.

Gallbladder attacks during pregnancy are most frequent in older multiparous women during the late stages of pregnancy. The symptoms are epigastric discomfort, colic, nausea, and vomiting. The incidence of acute cholecystitis ranges from 1 to 6 per 10,000 pregnant women. The most difficult diagnoses to exclude are appendicitis and acute pyelonephritis. Complications of acute cholecystitis are rare, however, obstructive jaundice develops in 7% of cases.

Gray scale ultrasonography is the preferred method of identifying gallstones in the pregnant patient. In selected cases an oral cholecystogram or other examinations necessitating radiation exposure may be indicated depending on the individual patient's clinical findings and the stage of the pregnancy.

The initial management of pregnant patients with acute cholecystitis should be medical and include restriction of oral intake, relief of pain with Demerol, and the administration of appropriate antibiotics. In uncomplicated cases, fetal loss is approximately 5% and the maternal mortality is the same as in nonpregnant women. When cholecystitis is complicated by pancreatitis, cholangitis, or rupture of the gallbladder, the fetal loss may be as high as 60% and the maternal mortality as great as 15%. (28)

Inflammatory Bowel Disease

Granulomatous Colitis (Crohn's Disease)

Granulomatous enterocolitis is a disease which most commonly affects young people, especially females. (29) It is commonly observed in Jews and in the northern United States, Canada, and western Europe. It is very uncommon in blacks and Orientals and in the southern United States and eastern Europe.

Granulomatous enterocolitis usually involves the distal part of the ileum and colon, although it may be found in any part or all of the GI tract. The etiology is unknown. A familiar pattern has been described. The inflammatory process starts in the mucosa but extends through the entire wall. The mucosa has a granulomatous appearance with ulcerations which give rise to the development of fistulae. The wall of the bowel and the mesentery are thickened and edematous. The fat of the mesentery extends to cover a portion of the wall of the intestine. Normal segments between diseased areas are called "skip" areas and are common in the small intestine. Perianal complications such as abscess or fistula may appear before symptoms of intestinal disease. Other complications include fistula between segments of intestine, and from diseased bowel to other organs or the skin surface. Marked narrowing of the lumen of the ileum, the "string sign," produced by marked thickening of the wall of the bowel, may produce obstruction. Bleeding from Crohn's disease of the small intestine is rare but bleeding from granulomatous colitis is common.

Crohn's disease commonly appears during the fertile age of the woman. A few patients develop symptoms during pregnancy but most pregnant patients with Crohn's disease have had symptoms prior to becoming pregnant. Most data suggests that only 13% to 15% of women with quiescent or mild Crohn's disease will have an exacerbation of their illness during pregnancy. However, women with active disease at the time of conception experience moderate to severe symptoms during pregnancy. For both groups exacerbation during the early postpartum period is common. This may be the result of the reduction in steroid production which follows delivery. (30)

It is important to recognize the symptoms as early as possible and begin treatment before the disease becomes severe or uncontrollable. Diffuse, persistent abdominal pain when accompanied by diarrhea makes the diagnosis likely. Since pregnant women tend to be constipated, diarrhea should rouse suspicion as should loss of weight despite an increase in food intake. Endoscopy of the rectum may provide the diagnosis. If not, the physician must presume the diagnosis and proceed with treatment or obtain additional diagnostic tests. Therapy consists of a nonirritating diet, corticosteroids, and sulfasalazine (Azulfindine). If the patient's oral intake is inadequate, hyperalimentation in the hospital or at home will be necessary to provide adequate maternal and fetal nutrition. (31) Fat emulsions are not recommended because of the development of postinfusion ketonemia and fatty infiltration of the placenta which may cause complications during pregnancy.

Administration of corticosteroids may control symptoms but the drug does cross the placenta. Most studies suggest the administration of cortisone is not associated with an increased risk of abortion or congenital malformation. Still, when Crohn's disease is severe, requiring steroids and sulfasalazine, then the incidence of abortion, stillbirths, and other complications is higher than in the normal population. (33)

Indications for operation for Crohn's disease include small bowel obstruction, abscess formation, free perforation, massive bleeding, or severe symptoms from well-localized disease not responding to medical therapy. The decision for operation should be made before the condition of the patient threatens the life of the mother and the fetus. Diseased segments of bowel should be removed if indicated and if possible. Operations which bypass diseased intestine should be avoided. Women with Crohn's disease who are considering pregnancy must be counseled regarding the risks.

Ulcerative Colitis

Ulcerative colitis is an inflammatory bowel disease which involves the mucosa of the colon and rectum. (34,35) The peak age of inset is between 20 and 40 years and it occurs more commonly in women than men. General observations suggest pregnancy does not affect the course of colitis. The reverse, the effect of ulcerative colitis on pregnancy, appears to be nonspecific. The percentage of normal deliveries, the number of therapeutic and spontaneous abortions, the percentage of stillbirths, premature babies, congenital abnormalities, and perinatal mortality were found to be the same as in the normal woman. (36)

The diagnosis of ulcerative colitis during pregnancy is best made by proctosigmoidiscopy and/or colonscopy rather than barium enema, thus avoiding the risks of radiation. The treatment of ulcerative colitis is similar to that of Crohn's disease with the principle medications being Azulfadine and cortisone. Indications for operation include (1) failure to control severe symptoms with medical management, (2) perforation of the colon, and (3) toxic megacolon. These complications are rare, but threaten both mother and fetus. When operation is indicated there must not be a delay.

Anorectal Disorders

These disorders are among the more common complications seen during pregnancy and usually appear in the last trimester. The enlarged gravid uterus and constipation are the two major causes.

Hemorrhoids

Hemorrhoids are enlarged veins which may cause unpleasant symptoms and complicate pregnancy. If they originate from the superior hemorrhoidal plexus, they are called internal hemorrhoids and are located above the anorectal line. Those from the inferior hemorrhoidal plexus are called external hemorrhoids and are located below the anorectal line in or outside the anal canal. The etiology is controversial. The traditional theory is that increased pressure in the pelvis obstructs the venous system, causing dilatation of the veins. The effect of constipation and the resulting straining to defecate increases the venous distention. Another theory suggests arteriovenous communications around the rectum are responsible for the development of hemorrhoids. A finding which supports the latter theory is the bright red color of the blood seen where hemorrhoids bleed. Finally, there may be a partial prolapse of the distal rectum and this, in combination with fibrous bands of the internal sphincter, produces partial obstruction of the hemorrhoidal plexus which causes venous distention and the development of the hemorrhoids. When studies by light microscopy hemorrhoidal views show atrophy of the adventitia and media.

Hemorrhoids may appear during pregnancy or be aggravated by pregnancy. If present prior to pregnancy they gradually increase in size during pregnancy and show marked diminution in size after delivery. Itching and pain, most severe when the patient is sitting, are the main symptoms. Bleeding usually is intermittent and associated with defecation. It is unusual for anemia to result from henorrhoidal bleeding. Severe pain and the appearance of a hard lump indicates thrombosis of an external hemorrhoid. If the thrombosis remains untreated, the mucosa which covers the thrombosed hemorrhoids may undergo necrosis resulting in an ulcer. Perirectal infections and/or fistula may occur as secondary complications. Occasionally a patient with severe constipation may prolapse the internal hemorrhoidal plexus and the rectal mucosa through the rectal sphincter resulting in marked edema, pain, and possible necrosis of tissue.

Treatment

Most hemorrhoids respond well to sitz baths, a low residual diet, bulk laxatives, and the application of a witch hazel preparation. Prolapsed hemorrhoids may require manipulation and reduction and/or the application of ice. Thrombosed external hemorrhoids respond well to evacuation of the clot and sitz baths. Operation is rarely required during pregnancy. The application of rubber bands and injection of sclerosing solutions may be employed in selected patients but medical management is best while the patient is pregnant.

Other Anal-Rectal Disorders

Fissure-in-ano, anal abscesses, cryptitis, papilitis, and fistula in-ano occur all too often during pregnancy. All these disorders have similar symptoms: pain, pruritis with a small amount of bleeding, and fever when an infection exists. Most of these disorders respond well to medical treatment. Operations for these disorders during pregnancy should ordinarily be limited to drainage of abscesses. Anal condylomas may be treated with local application of 25% podophyllum or may be removed surgically by cryosurgery or fulguration.

Hepatic Cirrhosis With Portal Hypertension

The two major complications of hepatic cirrhosis are upper GI bleeding and hepatic failure. Upper GI bleeding can occur from rupture of esophageal or gastric varices, gastric or duodenal ulcer, or acute hemorrhagic gastritis. In patients with cirrhosis, bleeding from a gastric or duodenal ulcer or acute hemorrhagic gastritis is as common as bleeding from gastro-esophageal varices.

Physiological changes during pregnancy which may cause complications in cirrhotic patients include:

1. Increased intra-abdominal pressure by the enlarged uterus

2. Increased splanchnic blood flow

3. Contractions of the diaphragm (37, 38)

4. Gastroesophageal reflex resulting in esophagitis

5. The stress during vaginal delivery which is found to increase the pressure of the portal vein in normal women

Pregnant women with portal hypertension are at increased risk of bleeding from the gastroesophageal varices during the second half of pregnancy, and the risk of bleeding increases with each subsequent pregnancy. (39-42)

Portal hypertension in itself has no adverse effect upon pregnancy. (43) Women with extrahepatic obstruction of the portal vein and compensated liver disease have an abortion rate similar to that of the general population. (44-47) In contrast, women with compromised hepatic function have an increased incidence of abortion (17. 5%). (48) Premature termination of pregnancy and perinatal mortality are distinctly higher in patients with jaundice and severe liver disease.

Cancer of the Gastrointestinal Tract During Pregnancy

Cancer of the gastrointestinal tract is extremely rare during pregnancy. The incidence is approximately 1:50,000 to 1:100,000. The reasons for this are twofold. First, gastrointestinal cancer is more frequent in males (with the exception of colorectal cancer where the percentages are almost equal in each sex). Secondly, this disease appears in an age group older than the childbearing years.

The symptoms of gastrointestinal malignancy are similar to those of pregnancy: persistent abdominal cramps, constipation, increased flatulence, vomiting, rectal bleeding, and weight loss are common. Whenever the etiology of these symptoms is in question, the gastrointestinal tract should be studied. The choice of endoscopy or barium contrast studies must be determined by the symptoms and the stage of pregnancy. Early operation is mandatory. The general approach is to treat the tumor and "ignore" the pregnancy.

Cancer of the Stomach

Gastric carcinoma has decreased steadily over the last two decades in the United States and Europe. However, its incidence remains high in Japan, Chili, Iceland, Finland, and China. It is most common in lower socio-economic groups. Fortunately, the incidence of gastric carcinoma is extremely low in the pregnant population, even in those countries where the incidence is high. (49) Gastric cancer is a disease of middle and late life and of males.

Endoscopy is the examination of choice for investigating possible stomach disorders, since it allows direct visualization and biopsy and avoids the risk of radiation. (50)

The treatment of gastric carcinoma is operation.

Tumors of the Small Bowel

There are a wide variety of benign and malignant tumors of the small bowel, although the overall incidence of these tumors is low. Common symptoms include cramping, abdominal pain, weight loss, and vomiting. Diagnosis, if made in advance of operation, is usually made by barium study of the small intestine. The exception is carcinoid tumors. Their presence may be detected by finding increased levels of 5 hydroxyindoleacetic acid in the urine.

Operation is the treatment of choice. Pregnancy is interrupted if obstetrical reasons warrant it or if the uterus is grossly infiltrated by the tumor. In most cases, the pregnancy is saved. Caesarean section is recommended if the fetus is viable.

Cancer of the Colon

Carcinoma of the colon is quite rare during pregnancy; an incidence of 0.002%. Most colorectal carcinomas are adenocarcinomas and have the same anatomical distribution as in the nonpregnant woman (57% rectal, 20% in the sigmoid colon, and 33% in other segments of the colon). Most pregnant women with carcinoma of the colon are between 35 and 40 years of age. (51) A history of premalignant disease of the colon such as inflammatory bowel disease, Gardner's syndrome, villous adenomas, or familial polyposis is found in 25%-30% of these patients. (52,53)

Symptoms are similar to those experienced by nonpregnant women. There may be early complaints of mild diffuse abdominal pain, distention, nausea, vomiting, and constipation. Later, more alarming symptoms occur such as rectal bleeding, vomiting, weakness, and weight loss. Weight loss is a symptom that should alert the physician, since during normal pregnancy a weight gain is expected.

Since most tumors are located in the rectum and sigmoid colon, digital examination of the rectum, proctosigmoidoscopy, and colonoscopy should be done whenever symptoms suggest a disorder of the colon or rectum.

The prognosis for patients with carcinoma of the colon during pregnancy is poor. The diagnosis is made late and extensive metastatic tumor is often present at the time of operation. In the first half of pregnancy, the operation is the same as for the nonpregnant patient. In the third trimester, if a viable fetus exists, an elective caesarean section should be performed. (54)

The bowel resection should be done at the same time as the caesarean section if the patient's condition allows. If the tumor is discovered close to the time of labor, a vaginal delivery may be followed by a bowel resection 2-4 weeks later. Chemotherapy and radiotherapy are better avoided during pregnancy, especially in the first trimester because of the teratogenic effects on the fetus. (55)

REFERENCES

1. Benson, RC. Current Obstetrics and Gynecologic Diagnosis and Treatment, 3rd ed. Lange Medical Publications, Los Altos, California, 1980.

2. Barber, HRK, and Graber, EA. Surgical Disease in Pregnancy. W. B. Saunders Co. , Philadelphia, 1974.

3. Seymour, CA, and Chadwick, VS. Liver and gastrointestinal function in pregnancy. Postgrad. Med. J. , 55(643): 343-356, 1979.

4. Sherlock, S. Diseases of the Liver and Biliary System. Oxford, Blackwell Scientific Publications, 1975, pp. 390-424.

5. Vender, RJ. Abdominal pain during pregnancy: A patient with Crohn's disease. Medi. Grand Rounds, 1(1):25-35, 1982.

6. Clement, PB. Perforation of the sigmoid colon during pregnancy: A rare complication of endometriosis: Case report. Br. J. Gynaecol. , 84(7):548-550, 1977.

7. Munro, A, and Jones, PF. Abdominal surgical emergencies in the puerperium. Br. Med. J. , 4:691-694, 1975.

8. Prust, FE, and Kumar, GK. Massive colonic bleeding and oral contraceptive "pills." Am. J. Gynecol. , 125(5):695-698, 1971.

9. Semchyshyn, S. Gastrointestinal hemorrhage in peurperium of pre-eclamptic patients who received glucocorticoid therapy. Am. J. Obstet. Gynecol., 139(2):217-218, 1981.

10. Wexler, P. Postpartum massive lower gastrointestinal bleeding. J. Rocky Mt. Med. , 74(1):33-34, 1977.

11. Deborja, C, Calem, WS, and Pochaczevski, R. Bleeding duodenal ulcer during pregnancy. NY State J. Med. , 71(8):876-879, 1971.

12. Becker-Anderson, H, et al. Peptic ulcer in pregnancy. Report of two cases of surgically treated bleeding duodenal ulcer. Acta Obstet. Gynec. Scand. , 50:391-395, 1971.

13. Babaknia, A, et al. Appendicitis during pregnancy. Am. J. Obstet. Gynecol. , 50(1):40-44, 1977.

14. Cunningham, FG, and McCubbin, JH. Appendicitis complicating pregnancy. J. Obstet. Gynec. , 45(4):415-420, 1975.

15. Farquharson, RG. Acute appendicitis in pregnancy. Scott Med. J. , 25:36-38, 1980.

16. Hasselgren, P. Acute pancreatitis in pregnancy. Acta Chir. Scand. , 146:297-299, 1980.

17. Gomez, A, and Wood, M. Acute appendicitis during pregnancy. Am. J. Surg. , 137:180-183, 1979.

18. Mohammed, JA, and Oxorn, H. Appendicitis in pregnancy. Can. Med. Assoc. , 112(1187):199-201, 1975.

19. McComb, P, and Laimon, H. Appendicitis complicating pregnancy. Can. J. Surg. , 23(1):92-94, 1980.

20. Townsend, JM, and Greiss, FC. Appendicitis in pregnancy. South. Med. J. , 69(9):1161-1163, 1976.

21. Coughlan, BM, and O'Herlihy, C. Acute intestinal obstruction during pregnancy. J-R Coll. Surg. Edinb. , 23(3):175-177, 1978.

22. Thomford, NR, et al. Appendectomy during pregnancy. Surg. Gynec. Obstet. , 129:489-492, 1969.

23. Hill, LM, Symmonds, RE. Small bowel obstruction in pregnancy: A review and report of four cases. Am. J. Obstet. Gynecol. , 49(2):170-173, 1977.

24. Acosta, JM, Pelligrini, MD, and Skinner, DB. Etiology and pathogenesis of acute biliary pancreatitis. Surgery, 88(1):118-125, 1980.

25. Burrow, GN, and Ferris, FT. Medical Complications During Pregnancy. W. B. Saunders Co. , Philadelphia, 1975.

26. Van Thiel, DH, et al. Heartburn of pregnancy. Gastroenterology, 72:666-668, 1977.

27. Braverman, DZ. Effects of pregnancy and contraceptive steroids on gallbladder function. N. Engl. J. Med. , 302(7):362-369, 1980.

28. Chaimoff, C, Dintsman, M, and Goldman, J. Rupture of the gallbladder in pregnancy with massive intraperitoneal hemorrhage. Int. Surg. , 58(10):741, 1973.

29. Donaldson, LB. Crohn's disease: "Its gynecologic aspect. " Am. J. Obstet. Gynecol. , 131(2):196-202, 1978.

30. Homan, WP, and Thorbjarnarson, B. Crohn disease and pregnancy. Arch Surg. , 111:545-547, 1978.

31. Cox, KL, Byrne, WJ, and Ament, ME. Home total parenteral nutrition during pregnancy: A case report. J. Parenteral Enteral. Nutrition, 5(3):246-249, 1981.

32. Moghdam, M, et al. The course of inflammatory bowel disease during pregnancy and postpartum. Am. J. Gastroenterol. , 75(4):265-269, 1981.

33. Moghdam, M, et al. Pregnancy in inflammatory bowel disease. Effect of sulfasalazine and corticosteroids on fetal outcome. Gastroenterology, 80(1):72-76, 1981.

34. Ganchrow, MI, and Benjamin, H. Inflammatory colorectal disease and pregnancy: Report of a case. Dis. Colon Rectum, 18(8):706-709, 1975.

35. Willoughby, CP, and Truelove, SC. Ulcerative colitis and pregnancy. Gut, 21(6):469-474, 1980.

36. Levy, N, Roisman, I, and Teodor, I. Ulcerative colitis in pregnancy in Israel. Dis. Colon Rectum, 24(5):351-354, 1981.

37. Palmer, ED. Effect of Valvalva's maneuver on portal pressure. Am. J. Sci. , 242:243, 1961.

38. Palmer, ED. Effect of Valsalva's maneuver on portal pressure. Am. J. Sci. , 227:661, 1974.

39. Evans, IM, Hoyuen, B, and Anderson, FH. Bleeding esophageal varices in pregnancy. Obstet. Gynecol. , 40(3): 377-380, 1972.

40. Salam, AA, and Warren, WD. Distal splenorenal shunt for the treatment of variceal bleeding during pregnancy. Arch Surg. , 105(4):643-644, 1972.

41. Cheng, YS. Pregnancy in liver cirrhosis and/or portal hypertension. Am. J. Obstet. Gynecol. , 128(7):812-822, 1977.

42. Whelton, MJ, and Sherlock, S. Pregnancy in patients with hepatic cirrhosis. Lancet, 2:995-999, 1968.

43. Niven, P, Williams, D, and Zeegren, R. Pregnancy following the surgical treatment of portal hypertension. Am. J. Obstet. Gynecol. , 110(8):1100-1112, 1971.

44. Donaldson, LB, and Plant, RK. Pregnancy complicated by extrahepatic portal hypertension: Review of literature and report of two cases. Am. J. Obstet. Gynecol. , 110(2): 255-264, 1975.

45. Wellborn, WR, Greiss, Jr. , FC, and Johnston, FR. Pregnancy following esophagectomy for bleeding varices in a patient with extrahepatic portal hypertension. Am. J. Obstet. Gynecol. , 117(2):181-183, 1973.

46. O'Leary, JA, and Bepko, Jr. , FJ. Portacaval shunt performed during pregnancy. Obstet. Gynecol. , 20:243-246, 1982.

47. Reisman, TM, and O'Leary, JA. Portacaval shunt performed during pregnancy. A case report. Obstet. Gynecol. , 37(2):253-254, 1971.

48. Varma, RR, et al. Pregnancy in cirrhotic and noncirrhotic portal hypertension. Obstet. Gynecol. , 50(2):217-222, 1977.

49. Sims, EH, et al. Obstructing gastric carcinoma complicating pregnancy. J. Natl. Med. Assoc. , 72(1):21-23, 1980.

50. Duckler, L, and Cohen, HR. Hyperemesis gravidarum with gastric carcinoma. Obstet. Gynecol. , 45(3):348-349, 1975.

51. Girard, RM, Lamarche, J, and Baillot, R. Carcinoma of the colon associated with pregnancy. Report of a case. Dis. Colon Rectum, 24(6):473-475, 1981.

52. Green, LK, Harris, RE, and Massey, FM. Cancer of the colon during pregnancy. A review of the literature and report of a case associated with ulcerative colitis. Obstet. Gynecol. , 46(4):480-483, 1975.

53. Schwartz, ML, and Beecham, JE. Villous adenoma of the rectum diagnosed during labor. Obstet. Gynecol. , 50(1 suppl.):7s-9sm, 1977.

54. Ovigstad, E, and Sande, HA. Carcinoma of the colon in pregnancy. Ann. Chir. Gynaecol. , 68(3):98-99, 1979.

55. Stephens, JD, et al. Multiple congenital anomalies in a fetus exposed to 5-fluorouracil during the first trimester. Am. J. Obstet. Gynecol. , 137(6):747-749, 1980.

56. Montgomery, WH, and Miller, FC. Pancreatitis and pregnancy. Obstet. Gynecol. 35:658-664, 1970.

Chapter 6

UROLOGIC PROBLEMS OF THE PREGNANT PATIENT

Steven H. Selman, M.D.

EMBRYOLOGIC AND ANATOMIC CONSIDERATIONS

The anatomic relationships between the urologic and reproductive systems are a result of their embryologic origin. (1-3) During early female fetal development, the mullerian ducts (paramesonephric ducts) fuse to form the uterovaginal canal, from which the fallopian tubes, uterus, and upper two-thirds of the vagina arise. The lower vagina and urethra develop from the pelvic portion of the urogenital sinus, maintaining throughout life an intimate relationship separated by loose connective tissue in the upper urethra but bound to one another by fusion of their fascia into a single dense layer in the lower urethra.

The Wolffian ducts (mesonephric ducts) enter the urogenital sinus adjacent to the fused mullerian ducts but regress in the female fetus after giving rise to the ureters. The pelvic portion of the ureter is accompanied by the uterine artery until it passes below the root of the broad ligament, where it passes below the artery lying about 2 cm lateral to the cervix above the lateral fornix of the vagina before inserting into the trigone of the bladder. The body of the bladder develops from the urogenital sinus directly anterior to the developing uterus. Both maintain an extraperitoneal location as contiguous organs deep within the bony pelvis separated by a fold of peritoneum on their opposing surfaces which forms the vesico-uterine pouch.

The metanephros originates at the level of the upper sacral segments but ascends out of the pelvis as the fetus elongates. Arrest in this ascent will result in an ectopic kidney.

PHYSIOLOGIC CHANGES OF PREGNANCY

The urinary tract can be divided into (1) an upper tract, kidneys, and ureters, responsible for the production and transport of urine, and (2) a lower tract, bladder and urethra, responsible for urinary storage and evacuation. Both upper and lower systems undergo physiologic changes during pregnancy.

Renal

The initial step in the formation of urine is glomerular filtration. Most investigators have reported that the renal plasma flow and glomerular filtration increase by at least 30 to 40% during the first trimester of pregnancy(4) and that this is maintained until term. As GFR increases, serum creatinine and blood urea nitrogen decrease. Despite an increase in GFR, total body water and sodium increase as pregnancy advances. (5) This results in part from an increase in tubular reabsorption of sodium and water. Sodium reabsorption is partially controlled by the renin-angiotensin-aldosterone system, which is stimulated during pregnancy. (6) It should be noted that in spite of the increased activity in the renin-angiotensin-aldosterone system, blood pressure usually drops during pregnancy. Renal tubular changes of pregnancy are further seen in the increase in glycosuria during pregnancy. Glycosuria, which occurs frequently in pregnancy, results from an increased GFR and the relative inability of the kidney in those affected patients to raise the transfer maximum (T_M) of glucose. (7) The same mechanism probably underlies the physiologic proteinuria of pregnancy. The last steps in the formation of urine, urinary concentration and maintenance of acid-base balance, are unimpaired during pregnancy. (8)

Ureteral

In most pregnancies there is a gradual development of hydronephrosis beginning between the sixth and tenth week of gestation, (9) this being most prominent in the first pregnancy. Ureteriectasis is more pronounced on the right but is limited in both ureters to the collecting system above the pelvic brim. The cause of hydronephrosis has been subject of considerable debate and investigation. (10-14) Most likely the effect is due to a combination of gradual compression from an enlarging uterus, decreased tonicity of the ureter, changes in the hormonal milieu, and the diuresis associated with increased GFR. In addition, dilatation of the ovarian veins which accompanies pregnancy contributes to ureteral dilatation, specifically the right ureter. The ovarian veins, which begin as a plexus deep in the pelvis, become a single vein at the level of L3 on the right and at the level of the renal pelvis on the left. The anatomic superimposition of the iliac vein, ureter, and ovarian vein on the right side accounts for lateralization of the "ovarian vein syndrome," which occurs when renal colic accompanies ureteral dilatation. (12)

As pregnancy progresses, the configuration of the ureterovesical angle changes. (13) The elevation of the trigone, lateral displacement of the ureters, and thickening of the muscular layers of the distal ureter predispose to ureterovesical reflux. (14) The incidence of reflux in the third trimester of pregnancy, as determined by chromoscopic methods, has been put at 3.4%. (15)

Bladder and Urethra

The lower urinary tract, bladder, and urethra perform as a highly integrated neuromuscular unit responsible for the storage of urine, maintenance of continence, and evacuation of urine. During pregnancy, frequency, nocturia, and incontinence are common. Several factors have been implicated: distortion of the vesicourethral angle as the uterus enlarges, an increased glomerular filtration rate which increases the rate of bladder filling, and an increase in mucosal sensitivity promoting bladder instability. (16, 17) These symptoms usually resolve after delivery. Urinary retention is an unusual problem during pregnancy but may be seen in the puerperium as a result of pelvic trauma incurred during labor and delivery.

RADIOGRAPHIC TECHNIQUES

Although the urologist has available an array of diagnostic tools that will delineate the site and extent of pathology in the genitourinary tract, these are employed only after weighing their risk to the fetus. Specifically, ionizing radiation potentially can induce congenital anomalies, carcinogenesis, and genetic defects in the fetus. Between the second and sixth week of gestation, the period of organogenesis, ionizing radiation is most hazardous. After the first trimester, congenital anomalies are unlikely to be induced by radiation. (18) That radiation can induce carcinogenesis is reflected by the high rates of leukemia found in survivors of atomic blasts as well as by reports of secondary cancers arising in patients treated with radiotherapy. (19)

Intravenous Pyelogram

The intravenous pyelogram (IVP) provides detailed information about the anatomy of the kidney and its collecting system. The typical intravenous pyelogram results in a radiation exposure level of 1 centigray, far less than the 50 centigray needed to cause radiation effect after the first trimester. However, it must be remembered the effects of radiation are dose dependent and that even small amounts of ionizing radiation are capable of inducing genetic mutations. Because of these concerns, techniques for decreasing radiation exposure should be employed during an IVP, i.e., use of prone rather than supine position, compression of bands around the maternal abdomen, collimating the beam, and using low kilovoltage. (20)

Ultrasound

As opposed to x-irradiation, ultrasonography poses no hazard to either mother or fetus. Ultrasonography provides accurate delineation of the anatomy of the kidney for both the parenchyma and the calyceal system. Ultrasonography is an especially sensitive technique for the detection of obstruction as reflected by calyceal dilatation. (21) In addition, ultrasonography has provided in utero diagnosis of fetal hydronephrosis as well as other congenital anomalies. (22)

Renal Scanning

The radioisotope renogram can provide both anatomic and physiologic data, although it is usually not as diagnostic as the standard intravenous pyelogram. The radiation risk from radioactive hippuran is small, on the order of 0.33 mrad to the mother and less to the fetus for a standard dose of 10 μCi hippuran. Of greater concern than hippuran radioactivity is the radiation exposure from the inorganic iodine which contaminates the hippuran preparation. This can be reduced with premedication of the mother with Lugol's solution. (23, 24) Information gleaned from the three phases of the renogram, the renal uptake, extraction, and drainage, can help assess renal function or the presence of obstruction.

Retrograde Pyelography

Retrograde pyelography can be employed where the previous methods have been nondiagnostic or when iodine sensitivity is present. As gestation progresses, however, retrograde ureteral catheterization becomes technically more demanding since the trigone is distorted by the enlarging uterus.

Antegrade Pyelography

Within the last decade there has been an explosion of reports in which closed diagnostic and therapeutic maneuvers have been performed through the combined use of fluoroscopy, ultrasonography, coaxial tomography, and percutaneous nephrostomy. A new discipline utilizing these modalities has been formed: "endourology."(25) Antegrade pyelography can be performed under local anesthesia and provides excellent radiographic detail of the urinary collecting system. If obstruction is present, percutaneous nephrostomy can provide an avenue for urinary tract decompression.

UROLOGIC DISEASE OF PREGNANCY

Urinary Tract Infection

Diminished renal function, anemia, prematurity, pre-eclampsia, congenital anomalies, and postpartum renal disease have all been linked to bacteriuria in pregnancy. (26-29) Whether these can, in fact, be attributed to urinary tract infection has been debated. (30, 31) However, prior to the antibiotic era acute pyelonephritis was associated with considerable morbidity and mortality. Since acute pyelonephritis of pregnancy will develop in 20-30% of patients with untreated bacteruria, the maintenance of sterile urine is an important prepartum goal. (32)

The most common urinary pathogen is E. coli, but the other enterobacteria, Proteus, Klebsiella, and Pseudomonas, also are found. The criteria for significant bacteriuria, $> 10^5$ organism/cc, has been well established. Lower counts do not rule out infection and should be repeated if indicated.

Urinary tract infections can be classified as simple, in which there are no underlying anatomic (e.g., obstructive) or pathologic (e.g., stone) processes; or as complex, in which these are present. Glycosuria and stasis of urine in ectatic ureters are conducive to infection. Patients with urinary tract infection can present with asymptomatic bacteruria, acute cystitis, or acute pyelonephritis. Treatment of asymptomatic bacteruria will decrease the number of patients developing acute pyelonephritis.

However, some patients will develop pyelonephritis without previously documented bacteruria. Patients with acute pyelonephritis should be hospitalized for vigorous antibiotic therapy. In patients with uncomplicated infection treatment is based on urinary culture and sensitivity. Familiarization with the potential side effects of urinary antibiotics is essential prior to the initiation of treatment. The sulfonamides are effective urinary antiseptics but should be given with caution near term because of their ability to displace bilirubin, causing kernicterus. (33) Tetracyclines have been associated with staining of deciduous teeth, while chloramphenicol used at term has been associated with a syndrome of vascular collapse, the so-called "gray baby syndrome."(34, 35) Most urinary tract infections of pregnancy will clear after seven to ten days of therapy. Repeat cultures should be obtained after completion of therapy. If there is recurrence, then suppressive therapy throughout pregnancy may be required. (36) It has been reported that bacteruria is often an indication of underlying chronic renal disease and that these patients deserve close follow-up. (28)

Congenital Problems

Pregnancy, unfortunately, does not confer immunity from the congenital, inflammatory, and neoplastic diseases of the urinary tract. Of the congenital anomalies, the ectopic pelvic kidney poses the greatest threat to the normal progression of labor and when it occurs is an indication for caesarean section. However, if the kidney lies outside the confines of the true pelvis, a vaginal delivery can be anticipated. Extrophy of the bladder is a relatively uncommon urologic congenital anomaly occurring 1 in 50, 000 births. Many of these patients have undergone a previous urinary diversion. The most common problem in pregnant patients with a history of extrophy is prolapse of the uterus and cervix. (37) Delivery should be vaginal if prolapse proceeds labor, while those who do not have significant prolapse prior to delivery should have caesarean section. (38, 39) Deliveries can be further complicated by a 25% malpresentation. The supravesical urinary diversion either for extrophy or other reasons does not appear to increase maternal risk during pregnancy. (40)

Renal Abscess

Uncomplicated pyelonephritis generally can be managed with intravenous antibiotics. Failure to respond to conservative treatment should arouse suspicion of a renal abscess and prompt further investigation. If detected, a renal abscess may require incision and drainage for adequate treatment, although recent reports of nonoperative management with percutaneous drainage are appealing. (41)

Stone Disease

Although urinary stone disease does not occur with increased frequency in the pregnant patient, diagnosis is made more difficult by the desire to minimize the radiation exposure to the fetus. (42) Signs and symptoms are similar to those found in the nongravid state: colic, nausea, and hematuria. If suspected, diagnosis can usually be confirmed with a plain abdominal film and a single film taken 20 minutes after the intravenous injection of contrast. Most stones less than 0.5 cm can be managed conservatively if not associated with high-grade obstruction or significant fever. Obstruction accompanied by infection requires prompt drainage. Obstruction can be relieved through retrograde ureteral catheterization, basket retrieval for lower ureteral stones and, if needed, percutaneous nephrostomy. Occasionally retrograde catheterization may push an obstructing ureteral calculus back into the renal pelvis. Recurrent obstruction at the ureteropelvic junction from a stone in the renal pelvis can be prevented through the use of self-retaining stents. (43) In some cases temporary measures are unsuccessful and surgery is required. Although technically possible during any part of pregnancy, the preferred time for open ureteral is during the second trimester.

Neoplasms

Neoplasms of the urinary tract are unusual in the childbearing years. Renal cell carcinoma during pregnancy has been the topic of several reports. (44, 45) Diagnosis may be delayed since signs and symptoms are often masked or misinterpreted. Diagnosis can usually be made by a combination of ultrasonography and arteriography. The treatment is **surgical**. Discovery of carcinoma of the bladder is extremely rare during pregnancy. Treatment, as in the nongravid patient, is dependent on the stage of the disease.

Renovascular Disease

Renovascular problems may present during pregnancy. Rupture of an aneurysm of the renal artery during pregnancy can be life-threatening. Pregnancy predisposes these aneurysms to rupture so that elective resection prior to pregnancy is indicated. Successful repair of a ruptured renal artery aneurysm without nephrectomy has recently been reported. (46) Renovascular hypertension may be first discovered during pregnancy. Pharmacologic treatment remains the initial mode of therapy, but surgical correction if necessary has been reported. (47)

Other Problems

Several unusual urologic problems have been associated with pregnancy. One problem, acute hydronephrosis of pregnancy, can lead to anuria or may be complicated by rupture of the kidney. (48, 49) Both are uncommon and both may be further complicated by massive renal hemorrhage. (50)

UROLOGIC INJURIES OF LABOR AND DELIVERY

Significant urologic trauma rarely accompanies routine vaginal delivery. However, as parity increases, partial inversion of the bladder through the urethera at the time of the delivery may occur. This usually can be managed through manual reduction. Occasionally the trauma of normal labor and episiotomy may create sufficient perineal discomfort to cause skeletal muscle spasm with resultant urinary retention. Short-term bladder catheterization will alleviate the problem.

Bladder Injury

In complicated labor and delivery there is a rise in urologic injury. The close proximity of the uterus to bladder places the bladder at the risk of injury should uterine rupture occur. (51) Vesico-vaginal fistula have resulted from prolonged, disproportionate labor and from the incorrect application of mid forceps, especially Kielland or Barton forceps. (52) Low transverse cervical incision for caesarean section also can injure the bladder if care is not taken to sweep the vesical reflection anteriorly. Nonsurgically created vesico-vaginal fistula typically involve the proximal urethra or bladder base below the ureteral orifices, while those of surgical origin arise above the trigone. The latter are categorized as either vesico-vaginal-cervical or vesico-cervical.

If injury to the bladder is recognized at the time of surgery, repair should be undertaken immediately. The bladder should be closed in layers (mucosa, muscular, and seromuscular) with absorbable suture material. Likewise, fistula occurring after prolonged or disproportionate labor may be attacked immediately, although local edema may make tissue approximation difficult. When fistula are first recognized by the appearance of urinary leakage from the vagina in the puerperium, repair should be delayed until the local tissue reaction has subsided. This usually necessitates a two- to three-month delay. There are, however, advocates of immediate repair of this problem.(53) Prior to surgical repair these patients should have an intravenous urogram, cystoscopy and, if necessary, retrograde pyelography to assess the site and extent of the fistula. These fistula can be approached vaginally or suprapubically. Successful repair depends upon complete separation of the edges of the bladder from the vagina.(54) Peritoneum or omentum can be interposed between the vesical and vaginal closures as added protection from recurrence.

<u>Ureteral Injury</u>

The ureter also is at risk during complicated labor and delivery. The pelvic ureter descends close to the uterine cervix prior to its insertion in the trigone. The anatomic intimacy of these two structures accounts for the injuries seen after complicated vaginal delivery and occasionally after caesarean section.

The ureter may be compromised by closure of a cervical or vaginal laceration, especially when bleeding obscures suture placement. Kielland forceps have reportedly injured the lower ureter when perforation of the lower uterine segment occurs. Operative control of hemorrhage during emergency hysterectomy for uterine rupture, or control of bleeding into the broad ligament after a transverse lower uterine segment incision also can result in injury to the lower ureter. Ureteral injuries in these situations take the form of crush injury, ligation, or transection.

Treatment must be individualized, but in general transection or crush injury to the lower pelvic ureter recognized intraoperatively should be managed by ureteral reimplantation. If an extensive area of the lower ureter is damaged, the surgeon may need to employ a Boari flap or Psoas hitch to allow for a tension-free anastomosis. Delay in recognition can result in a septic course, which is best handled with proximal diversion allowing for resolution of the periureteral inflammatory process. Ligation of the ureter if recognized at the operating table may only require deligation, especially if surrounding tissue is included in the ligature. If ureteral ligation is recognized postoperatively, then removal should be done as quickly as possible. If it is removed within one week, chances of a successful outcome are good; between one and two weeks success is about 50%, and after

two weeks ureteral stricture will result. (55) A ligature placed
adjacent to the ureter without incorporating the wall but creating
angulation and obstruction at times can be corrected with the
placement of a ureteral stent. Untreated distal ureteral injury will invariably result in ureteral stricture or ureteral vaginal fistula.

RENAL TRANSPLANTATION

With the introduction of successful techniques for renal transplantation, fertility can be restored to patients with chronic
renal failure. These pregnancies require careful monitoring to
prevent compromise of graft, mother, or fetus. Hypertension,
increased proteinuria, and a 9% renal rejection rate have been
reported. Pre-eclampsia develops in up to 30% of these pregnancies, while prematurity ranges from 12 to 50%. (56, 57) Sur-
prisingly, immunosuppression does not appear to have a deleterious effect on the fetus since congenital anomalies are uncommon. (58) Dystocia resulting from the transplanted kidney
has not been a problem. Patients should be advised to wait at
least 18 months after transplantation before considering pregnancy and only then when they fulfill the criteria outlined by
Davidson (59):

1. Stature compatible with good obstetric outcome

2. No proteinuria

3. No significant hypertension

4. No evidence of renal rejection

5. No pelvi-calyceal distention

6. Plasma creatinine 2 mg/dl or less

7. Drug therapy: prednisone 15 mg/day or less and
    azathioprine 3 mg/kg/day or less

REFERENCES

1. Meuke, EC. The embryology of the urinary system. In Campbells' Urology. Philadelphia, W. B. Saunders Co., p. 1287, 1979.

2. Arey, LB. Developmental Anatomy, 7th ed. Philadelphia, W. B. Saunders Co., pp. 326-327, 1974.

3. Patten, BM. Human Embryology, McGraw-Hill, p. 473, 1968.

4. Sims, EA, and Krantz, KE. Serial studies of renal function during pregnancy and the puerperium in normal woman. J. Clin. Invest., 37:1764, 1958.

5. Kellerman, E. Renal control of electrolytes and acid-base balance during pregnancy. In The Kidney in Pregnancy, deAlvarey, RR (Ed.). New York, John Wiley & Sons, 1976.

6. Wilson, M, Morganti, AE, Zervoudakis, I, et al. Blood pressure, the renin aldosterone system, and sex steroids throughout normal pregnancy. Am. J. Med., 68:97, 1980.

7. Welsh, CW, and Sims, EA. The mechanisms of renal glycosuria in pregnancy. Diabetes, 9:363, 1960.

8. Rowe, JN, Brown, RS, and Epstein, FH. Physiology of the kidney in pregnancy. In Urology in Pregnancy, Freed, SZ, and Hurzig, N (Eds.). Baltimore, Williams and Wilkins, 1982.

9. Roberts, JA. Hydronephrosis of pregnancy. Urology, 8:1, 1976.

10. Bellina, JH, Dougharty, CM, and Michal, A. Pyeloureteral dilatation and pregnancy. Am. J. Obstet. Gynecol., 108:356, 1970.

11. Marchant, DJ. Effects of pregnancy and progestational agents on the urinary tract. Am. J. Obstet. Gynecol., 112:487, 1972.

12. Roberts, JA. The ovarian vein and hydronephrosis of pregnancy. Invest. Urol., 8:610, 1971.

13. Hofbauer, J. Structure and function of the ureter during pregnancy. J. Urol. 2:413, 1928.

14. Sala, NL, and Rubi, RA. Ureteral function in pregnant women. V. Incidence of vesicoureteral reflux and its effect upon ureteral contractility. Am. J. Obstet. Gynecol., 112:871, 1972.

15. Mattingly, RF. In Discussion of paper by Merchant, PJ, Effects of pregnancy and progestational agents on the urinary tract. Am. J. Obstet. Gynecol., 112:487, 1972.

16. Francis, WJA. Disturbance of bladder function in relation to pregnancy. J. Obstet. Gynecol. Br. Empire, 67:353, 1960.

17. Duncan, JW, and Seng, MI. Factors predisposing to pyelitis in pregnancy. Am. J. Obstet. Gynecol., 16:557. 1928.

18. Swartz, HM, and Reichling, BA. Hazards of radiation exposure for pregnant women. JAMA, 239:1907, 1978.

19. Kleinerman, RA, Curtis, RE, Borce, JD, Flannery, JT, and Fraumeni, JF. Second cancers following radiotherapy for cervical cancer. J.N.C.I. 69(5):1027, 1982.

20. Stern, WZ. Diagnostic imaging of the urinary tract in pregnancy. In Urology in Pregnancy, Freed, SZ, and Hurzig, N (Eds.). Baltimore, Williams and Wilkins, 1982.

21. Russell, JM, and Resnick, MI. Ultrasound in urology. Urol. Clinics N. Am., 6:2, 1979.

22. Kay, L, Lee, TG, and Tank, ES. Ultrasonographic diagnosis of fetal hydronephrosis in uretero. Urology, 13:286, 1979.

23. Wax, SH, and Rudolph, JH. The ^{131}I renogram in pregnancy. I. Safety. Obstet. Gynecol., 30:381, 1967.

24. Seltzer, R, Kerkiakes, JG, and Saenger, EI. Radiation exposure from radioisotopes in pediatrics. N. Engl. J. Med., 271:84, 1964.

25. Smith, AD. Endourology. Urol. Clinics N. Am., 9:1, 1982.

26. Williams, GL, Campbell, H, and Davies, KJ. Urinary concentrating ability in women with asymptomatic bacteuria in pregnancy. Br. Med. J., 3:212, 1969.

27. Monzon, DT, Armstrong, D, Pion, RJ, Deigh, R, and Hewitt, WL. Bacteruria during pregnancy. Am. J. Obstet. Gynecol., 85:511, 1963.

28. Kincaid-Smith, P, and Bullen, M. Bacteriuria in pregnancy. Lancet, 1:395, 1965.

29. Cunningham, FG, Morris, GD, and Michal, A. Acute pyelonephritis of pregnancy: A clinical review. Obstet. Gynecol., 42:112. 1973.

30. Kass, EH. Pyelonephritis and bacteriuria. Ann. Intern. Med., 56:46, 1962.

31. Turck, M, Goeffe, BS, and Petersdorf, RG. Bacteriuria of pregnancy. N. Engl. J. Med., 266:857, 1962.

32. Whalley, PJ. Bacteriuria of pregnancy. Am. J. Obstet., 97:723, 1967.

33. Odell, GB. Dissociation of bilirubin from albumin and its clinical implications. J. Pediatr., 55:268, 1959.

34. Wallman, IS, and Hilton, HB. Teeth pigmented by tetracycline. Lancet, 1:827-829, 1962.

35. Sutherland, JM. Fatal cardiovascular collapse of infants receiving large amounts of chloramphenicol. J. Dis. Child., 97:761, 1959.

36. Harris, RE, and Gilstrap, III, LC. Prevention of recurrent pyelonephritis during pregnancy. Obstet. Gynecol., 44:637, 1974.

37. Stanton, SL. Gynecological complications of epispadium and bladder extrophy. Am. J. Obstet. Gynecol., 119:749, 1974.

38. Krisiloff, M, Punchner, PJ, Treter, W, Macfarlane, MT, and Lattimer, JK. Pregnancy in women with bladder extrophy. J. Urol., 119:478, 1978.

39. Clemetson, C. Ectopic vesical and split pelvis. An account of pregnancy in a woman with treated ectopia vesicae and split pelvis, including a review of the literature. J. Obstet. Gynecol. Br. Empire, 65:973, 1958.

40. Kohler, FP. Management of pregnancy following lower urinary tract diversion. Am. J. Obstet. Gynecol., 97: 1149, 1967.

41. Finn, DJ, Palestrant, AM, and DeWolf, WC. Successful percutaneous management of renal abscess. J. Urol., 127:425, 1982.

42. Coe, FL, Parks, JH, and Lindheimer, MD. Nephrolithiasis during pregnancy. N. Engl. J. Med., 298:324, 1978.

43. Finney, RP. Experience with new double J ureteral catheter stents. J. Urol., 120:678, 1978.

44. Pelosi, M, Hung, CT, Langer, A, Khademi, M, and Harrigan, JT. Renal carcinoma in pregnancy. Obstet. Gynecol., 45:461, 1975.

45. Ney, C, Posner, AC, and Ehrlich, JC. Tubular adenoma of the kidney during pregnancy. Obstet. Gynecol., 37:267-276, 1971.

46. Love, WK, Robinette, MK, and Vernon, CP. Renal artery aneurysm rupture in pregnancy. J. Urol., 126:809, 1981.

47. Ito, Y, Falkinburg, N, Rogers, DT, and Martin, DC. Renal vascular hypertension in pregnancy: Problems in diagnosis and management. J. Urol., 108:9, 1972.

48. Schloss, WA, and Solom, KV. Acute hydronephrosis of pregnancy. J. Urol., 68:885, 1952.

49. Kolbusz, WE, and Carter, MF. Renal insufficiency in a solitary kidney secondary to hydronephrosis of pregnancy. J. Urol., 122:823, 1979.

50. Apperson, JW. Massive bleeding from hydronephrosis of pregnancy. J. Urol., 89:156, 1963.

51. Hassim, AM. Uterine rupture with extrusion of the fetus into the bladder. Int. Surg., 49:130, 1968.

52. Freed, SZ. Injury to the lower urinary tract resulting from pregnancy. In Urology in Pregnancy, Freed, SZ, and Hurzig, N (Eds.). Baltimore, London, Williams and Wilkins, 1982.

53. Persky, L, Herman, G, and Guerrier, K. Nondelay in vesico-vaginal fistula repair. Urology, 13:273, 1974.

54. Gray, PA. Obstetric vesicovaginal fistula. Am. J. Obstet. Gynecol., 107:898, 1970.

55. McDougal, WS, and Persky, L. Traumatic injuries of the genitourinary system. In International Perspectives in Urology, Vol. 1, Baltimore, London, Williams and Wilkins, 1981.

56. Rudolph, JE, Schweizer, RT, and Baitus, SA. Pregnancy in renal transplant patients -- a review. Transplantation, 27:26, 1979.

57. Rifle, G, and Traeger, J. Pregnancy after transplantation: An international survey. Transplant Proc. Suppl., 1:723, 1975.

58. Saarikoski, S, and Seppala, M. Immunosuppression during pregnancy: Transmission of azathioprine and its metabolites from the mother to the fetus. Am. J. Obstet. Gynecol., 115:1100, 1973.

59. Davison, JM, Lind, T, and Udall, PR. Planned pregnancy in a renal transplant recipient. Br. J. Obstet. Gynecol., 83:518, 1976.

Chapter 7

PERIPHERAL VASCULAR PROBLEMS DURING PREGNANCY

J. Robert Navarre, M.D.,

Of all the systems of the body, the vascular system (particularly the venous side) manifests widespread changes with the onset and progress of pregnancy. As a result of changes in the anatomy and physiology, there are marked alterations in its function, which provide the background for potential problems. These range from merely troublesome, as in superficial phlebitis, to the catastrophic situations, such as pulmonary embolism or disseminated intravascular coagulation (DIC).

Historically there has been an interest in the relationship between pregnancy and the afflictions of the veins, extending back to the period even prior to Harvey's description of the circulation. Those interested in venous problems pursued the effects of pregnancy and its possible relationship to venous difficulties. In the mid-sixteenth century, Marianus Sanctus Barolitanns(13) wrote that "child bearing and standing too much before kings" were the chief causes of varicose veins. In 1579, Ambroise Pare(7) stated that "women with child are commonly troubled by them (varicose veins) by reason of suppression of the menstrual evacuation."

Even after Harvey, in the seventeenth and eighteenth centuries, writers continued to promulgate the theory that menstrual blood collected in the legs during pregnancy, resulting in varicose veins and ulceration. This interest has continued down to the present day, with the obstetrician ever alert to these problems in regard to both prevention and recognition.

The circulation in pregnancy is affected for the most part on the venous side. The lower extremities are drained by the deep and superficial venous system. The deep system returns 90% of the blood, the length of the leg, to the level of the inguinal ligament. The superficial venous system drains and is responsible for collecting and channeling 10% of the blood for this distance. It mainly conveys the blood for short distances and then diverts it through the communicating veins to the deep venous system. Thus we refer to the gross unit of function, consisting of the superficial venous system, connected to the deep venous system by the communicating veins. This unit is dependent for its integrity upon the intraluminal valves, which channel the blood cephalad and deep (Figs. 7-1 and 7-2).

At the tissue level there is a similar balanced situation, with flow from the artery to the arterioles to the cellular level. There is a balance of flow between the hydrostatic force and the tissue pressure, with flow of fluid and nutrients out at the arterial end. Then, at the venous capillary side, the balance changes, and there is a flow of fluids, metabolites, and manufactured products into the venous channels for return to the right side of the heart. This is the microscopic unit of function (see Fig. 7-2).

These factors are altered to varying degrees during pregnancy by the increased pressure in the pelvis, secondary to venous flow.

Physiologically, there are three factors responsible for venous return. The role of the heart, for the most part is capacitance, apportioning the amount of blood on the venous and the arterial side. The changes in intracavitary pressure, pleural and abdominal, plus the peripheral pump mechanisms, are the major factors in venous return. With the decrease in intrathoracic pressure, secondary to diaphragmatic excursions, the blood is literally siphoned into the major thoracic veins. Conversely, anything promoting increased intra-abdominal pressure would decrease this effect. The peripheral muscles of the calf and thigh, with the valved venous sinuses and vascular channels, particularly in the leg, provide essential propulsion of the blood with each contraction during ambulation. With pregnancy, there are hormonal changes, hematologic changes, and even changes in blood volume that promote changes in flow and the clotting mechanism, often initiating the frequent complications of varicose veins and venous thrombosis.

Distention of the venous system, by a combination of increased circulating blood volume (plasma volume, increased varying from 630 to 1940 m, and red blood cell volume, increasing 30-40% (11-19) and the hormonal effects that occur early and last throughout pregnancy. This distention distorts and renders incompetent segments of the saphenous system (see Figs. 7-1 and 7-2), particularly in the patient with a

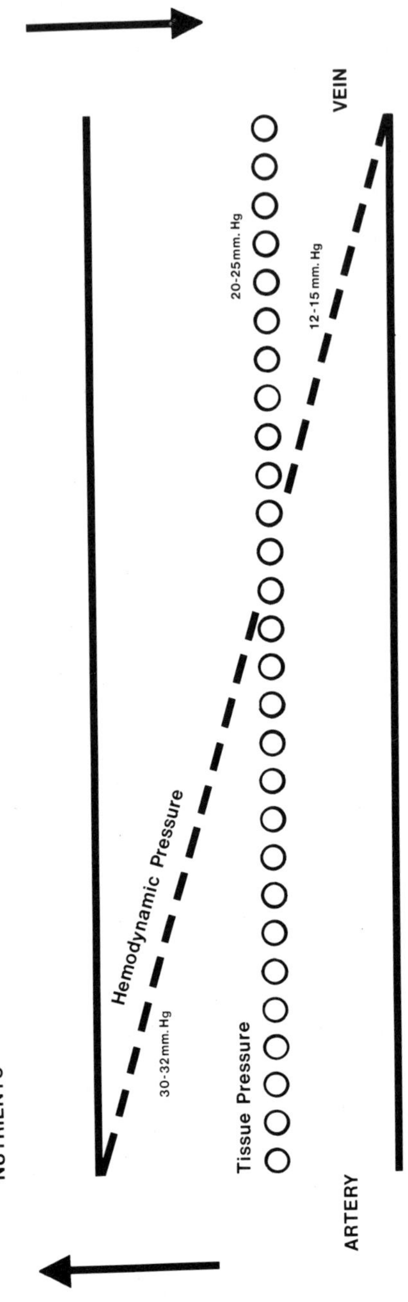

FIGURE 7-1. Gross unit of function.

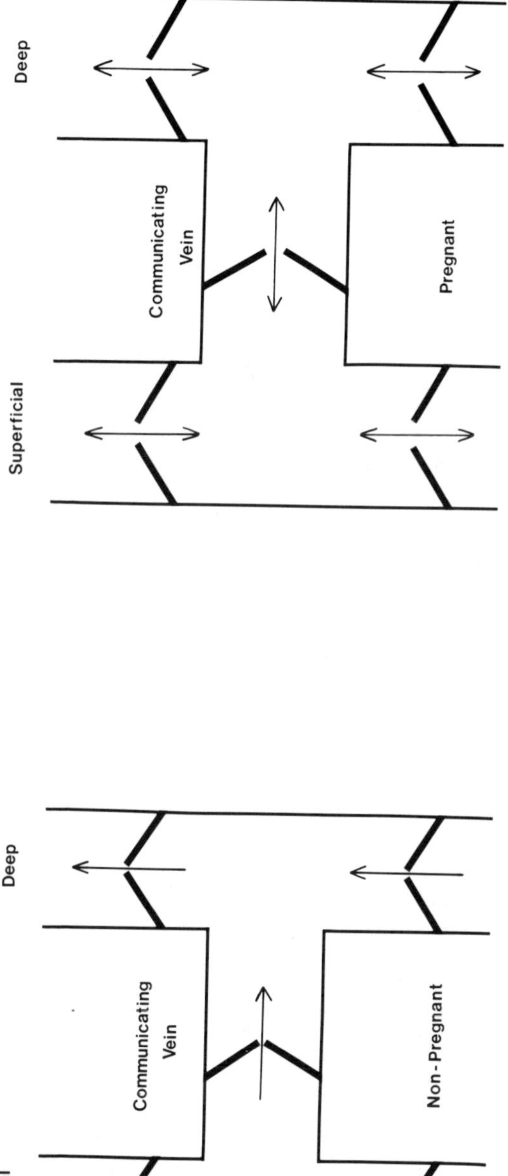

FIGURE 7-2. Microscopic unit of function.

congenitally decreased number of valves. Mechanically there is a large increase in pelvic flow, in addition to the obstructive effects of the uterus, particularly until it rises out of the pelvis in the latter stages of pregnancy. Functionally, pregnancy compromises to a certain degree the venous flow toward the right side of the heart by changes in the intra-abdominal pressure, particularly in the latter stages of pregnancy when the gravid uterus usurps a great portion of the abdominal cavity. The elevation of the diaphragm and resultant changes in excursion further compromise venous return. The peripheral pump mechanism functions less efficiently due to changes in muscular tone and the decreased activity of pregnancy.

Finally, there are changes in the coagulation mechanism that promote decreased clotting time. Some of the changes have been noted by Alexander. (3) Increase in Factor VII is noted in 80% of the gravid females, and the elevation of Factor X may be two to three times normal. Moseley and Kerstein indicated in a 1980 review (16) additional changes with rises in the fibrin split products, increase in the presence of clotting factors, and decrease in the fibrinolytic mechanisms. All these responses to pregnancy complicate and alter the functioning of the venous system. Venous distention and varicose veins are the early and most frequent manifestations of these alterations. In the patient with varicosities, there is aggravation of this previous existing state. In the individual with borderline competence or a congenitally deficient number of intraluminal valves, varicosities are produced.

VARICOSE VEINS

The symptoms of varicose veins are aching and fatigue, proportional to the time spent on the feet or with the feet in a dependent position. There is production or aggravation often of nocturnal "charley horses." The findings are limited usually to varying degrees of ankle edema, accumulating as the day progresses and relieved by elevation, and by the prominent distention of the superficial veins, with varying degrees of tortuosity. If pigmentation, ulcerations, or varices are present prior to pregnancy, they will, of course, be enhanced.

Treatment of the varicose veins is expectant and non-surgical. Elevation plus external support are the basic tenets of therapy at this time. Many of the patients with striking varicosities regain competence of the superficial system postpartum. However, the typical history is progression of these vacular deficits with subsequent pregnancies. Usually periodic elevations (midmorning and midafternoon with modest elevation of the foot of the bed at night) combined with elastic bandages or pressure gradient supports are sufficient to control the symptoms within tolerable limits.

Surgery at this stage is not advisable for a number of reasons. First, because of the lack of predictability of the future status of the dilated groups during pregnancy. Second, because of the compromise of careful deliberate surgery by the presence of the fetus. Third, because of risk to the fetus itself. If ligation and stripping is to be carried out, it would best be done on an elective basis, 8-12 weeks postpartum when all the alterations of pregnancy have terminated. Prior to this time there is a risk of complication secondary to the large dilated pelvic veins, on occasion containing bland thrombi.

Two subgroups of patients present during pregnancy: (1) the patient with labial varicosities and (2) the patient who has spider nevi. The patient with labial varices (7) has these as a result of a breakdown of the valves in the terminal portion of the iliac veins, just below the uterine veins. There is a large amount of pressure with reflection via the obturator and the internal pudendal veins to the labia, vagina, and posterior thighs. Surgery is usually ineffective. The use of a pressure gradient type of waist-high garment support, with the placement of sanitary pads to support the labia, is the most effective method of control. These groups of varices usually subside after delivery. If not, then surgical excision in the postpartum course may be indicated. Spider nevi or spider veins are unsightly and distressing. They have some hormonal dependence, but are not of frank pathological significance. They are grossly aggravated by pregnancy and are an indication for pressure gradient supports at the knee or thigh level. Patients should have these supports fitted in the first trimester of pregnancy, and they should be worn throughout.

Dysfunction of the arterial system is a rarity in pregnancy. Because of the age group, vasospastic disease is usually the only entity encountered. It is noteworthy that pregnant females have an increased flow in the digits of the upper extremities in particular during pregnancy. This is a reflection of the decreased peripheral resistance, probably secondary to progesteronal levels. Thus vasospastic disease (14-17) improves or becomes asymptomatic during pregnancy.

THROMBOSIS

In thrombosis, because of the changes associated with the gravid state, the factors in Virchow's triad are exacerbated to varying degrees such as changes in flow and in the wall of the vessel. By extension, coagulation factors are elevated such as in Factors VII and X and changes in the blood itself. Thus the problem with thrombosis is, varying from superficial to those with more lethal implications, deep venous thrombosis and disseminated intravascular coagulation.

Thrombosis occurs in 1:70(16) cases of pregnancy or post-delivery. The most frequent sites are the pelvic veins and the veins of the lower extremities, including the calf and tibial veins. Aaro in 1974(2) stated that in 32,000 pregnancies at the Mayo Clinic there was an incidence of superficial thrombophlebitis of 1:662 pregnancies antepartum and 1:95 postpartum. Deep venous thrombosis occurred in 1:1902 pregnancies antepartum and 1:668 postpartum.(1-2) Moseley and Kerstein(16) quote a survey in England and Wales from 1961 through 1966 in which there were 1300 maternal deaths. Pulmonary embolism was secondary only to abortion as the primary cause. In this same review by Moseley and Kerstein, the incidence of nonfetal pulmonary embolism in pregnancy and the puerperium varied from 0.27%(9) to 1.2%(18). Coon(6) and others documented the increased risk of thrombosis and its sequelae incidental to pregnancy.

Additional risk factors over and above the pregnancy are increased parity, age over 30, a history of previous venous problems (especially thromboembolic), prolonged labor or bedrest, and operative delivery, either a complicated forceps procedure or caesarean section.

Finnerty and McKay(8) in a series found pulmonary embolism and deep venous thrombosis (DVT) the same in all types of delivery by the vaginal route, 0.26%. However, those patients with caesarean section had an incidence of 0.66% per 100 deliveries. In their series they also note that patients with fetal thromboembolic episodes, 75% followed caesarean sections. Figures have improved, however. One of the most recent series indicated mortality from pulmonary embolism after caesarean section had fallen from 1.8 per 10,000 to 0.2 for vaginal deliveries as compared to 5.3 per 10,000 for caesarean sections and 0.9 per 10,000 vaginal deliveries from 1955 through 1957.(16)

The thrombus usually originates secondary to venous dilatation and begins in valve cusps and saccules of the dilated veins. (4) The left side is more frequently involved than the right. It is thought to be due to the stasis aggravated by compression of the left iliac vein by the right iliac artery at the promontory of the sacrum, where it crosses to form the confluence of the inferior vena cava.

SUPERFICIAL THROMBOPHLEBITIS

The patient with superficial thrombophlebitis presents typically with erythema, induration, and superficial tenderness, usually along the course of the saphenous branches. There is no ankle edema or fullness of the calves. The patient is usually more concerned about the implications of a "clot traveling" than actual discomfort. Examination usually reveals little beyond the aforementioned findings. The patient commonly has no edema or deep tenderness. The noninvasive laboratory, usually, is of great value in ruling out the possibility, by venous plethysmography, of any element of involvement of the deep venous system. Treatment is supportive with local heat, mild analgesics, and anti-inflammatory agents such as aspirin and a moderation of activities. In recalcitrant cases, it may be necessary to use anti-inflammatory agents such as phenylbutazone.

Surgery is rarely indicated except in the patient with a rapidly extending process on the medial aspect of the thigh, extending to the groin. If such a patient is nonresponsive to conservative treatment, interruption at the groin under local anesthesia is indicated. Such individuals have progressed to produce an extension to the saphenofemoral confluence and have been the source of pulmonary emboli or involvement of the deep venous system. In these patients no definitive ligation of the other branches or stripping is carried out. Three months after delivery, these patients should have ligation and stripping of the greater and lesser saphenous system with ligation of the incompetent communicating veins.

DEEP VENOUS THROMBOSIS

Deep venous thrombosis often presents with a paucity of symptoms. The complications of pulmonary embolism may well be the first indication of the presence of a clot in the deep venous system. Painless, unilateral edema or aching and fatigue of the extremities may be the only complaints. Examination grossly may reveal only borderline swelling of the limb and some tenderness between the heads of the gastrocnemius. We do not usually give credit to a "positive Homan's sign." This may be significant but is usually equivocal, even when performed in the proper manner. Application of the sphygmomanometer with gentle inflation will often reveal significant differentiation of tolerance for pressure between the two limbs. Once suspicion has been aroused, definitive delineation of the exact diagnosis is imperative because of the potential cata-

strophic implications and the necessity for planning a therapeutic regimen. The mainstay of screening and diagnosis is the
doppler venous examination and impedance plethysmography or
other types of venous plethysmography such as rheography.

Examination by the hand doppler is a valuable tool to the
obstetrician or those treating peripheral vascular disease. The
basic principle is examination of venous flow by the application
of the hand doppler to the groin over the common femoral vein.
Normally, with changes in expiration and inspiration, one should
hear rushes of venous blood beneath the doppler head, as a response to changes in intrathoracic and intra-abdominal pressure.
In addition to these, one should have augmentation of this flow
and sound with manual compression of the muscles of the thigh
and the calf, when the legs are placed in a moderately flexed
position.

Plethysmography is based on measuring the changes in the
volume of the limbs when the superficial venous return is obstructed. These changes can be measured in a number of
ways. We use the change of flow or impedence of a weak gal-
vanic current. This is known as impedance plethysmography
(IPG). Normally, there should be a rapid rise followed by a
rapid fall when the pressure is released. These volumetric
changes are plotted on a nomogram, and the values are rendered
as normal or abnormal. When a combination of venous doppler examination and venous plethysmography in an individual
with a clinical picture of deep venous thrombosis shows a positive doppler examination and a positive venous plethysmography
examination, the next procedure usually is phlebography. However, in the pregnant patient, even with shielding, there is
some implication for the fetus. In a study of 163 limbs at our
institution, we had a sensitivity of 96% with a specificity of 81%
with an incidence of false negative of 0.61%. This indicated a
high degree of accuracy with a very low degree of false nega-
tives (0.61%). Thus we feel secure in proceeding to therapy
without phlebography. In the postpartum patient, however, one
should proceed to definitive evaluation by phlebography which
rapidly and firmly establishes the diagnosis.

Therapy is directed at preventing progression and mobiliza-
tion of the clot. General measures include bedrest, elevation
of the foot of the bed, and local warm, moist packs. The use
of a bedside commode seems less likely to promote mobiliza-
tion of the clot by changing the intra-abdominal pressure than
a bedpan and thus is permitted. The patient is anticoagulated
by a continuous intravenous route. An initial bolus of 3000
units of heparin is given, and the patient is maintained on the
dose indicated by the activated partial thromboplastin times
(PTT). Usually 1200 units/hour is the starting dose. The PTT

is drawn every 12 hours until a therapeutic level is reached, two to three times the control, 50-70 minutes. Then, with daily monitoring of the PTT, this range is maintained for 7-10 days, depending on the clinical course and findings.

Additional monitoring of the patient by daily platelet counts is indicated. (20) **A small subset of patients on heparin therapy** do have heparin-induced thrombosis. When the heparin route is intravenous, the only warning sign may be the progressive thrombocytopenia. In such situations, heparin should be discontinued and appropriate studies done to delineate the process carried out. At the end of this time, if the patient is asymptomatic, she is fitted with pressure gradient supports to the lower extremities and ambulated. In the postpartum patient, consideration for oral anticoagulants may be indicated if the patient has had extensive involvement and edema. However, in the gravid patient, no oral anticoagulants are used because of the drug passing the placental barrier and being responsible on occasion for damage to the fetus.

Drugs(16) with a molecular weight of less than 1000 will pass the placental barrier. Heparin, with a molecular weight of 20, 000, does not cross the placental barrier. Warfarin, by crossing the placental barrier, can cause further aggravation of the already vitamin K-dependent clotting factors that are low in the fetus. (18) Birth defects, consisting of mental retardation, deafness, and blindness, have been recorded in infants whose mothers have had oral anticoagulants in the first trimester. (16) Women who have been on oral anticoagulants have an incidence of 15-18. 4% of fetal deaths, usually secondary to hemorrhage during or following delivery. Heparin has few side effects and can be rapidly reversed in the event of the onset of labor. Using heparin during the first trimester and switching to oral anticoagulants until just prior to delivery has been suggested but is not our current practice.

PHLEGMASIA ALBA DOLENS

Phlegmasia alba dolens was first reported by Wiseman in 1676. (7). It was subsequently described by Puzas(7) in 1759, and both believed this was due to excessive humors of the uterus and lactation. Finally, it was described in a more modern context by Davis in 1822(7) and by Trousseau in 1825. The syndrome is characterized by a pale, swollen, painful extremity of relatively sudden onset. There may be a decrease in the pedal pulses due to spasm from irritation of the adjacent iliac artery. It is often confused with arterial embolism, but the patient retains sensation, motor power, and the pain is much less severe.

The location of the thrombosis is at the iliac level. Very seldom do these patients experience embolization. Treatment consists of warm, moist packs, elevation, anticoagulation with heparin, and occasionally lumbar sympathetic block. On rare occasions venous thrombectomy may be required, and at least on one occasion in the past a patient who had not been treated promptly required arterial thrombectomy.

PHLEGMASIA CERULEA DOLENS

The other variant of deep venous thrombosis is phlegmasia cerulea dolens. This is characterized by a swollen, purple, painful limb, usually of massive degree. It is insidious in onset, and usually there are more grave implications than with phlegmasia alba dolens. The pathology consists of total infrainguinal venous thrombosis and more frequently gives rise to pulmonary embolism than does phelgmasia alba dolens. Inasmuch as there is no outlet for venous blood, there is no adequate arterial inflow and gangrene may result. This often has been referred to as paradoxical or venous gangrene. Treatment consists of elevation, anticoagulation, and warm, moist packs with careful observation. If the patient has not responded with a decrease in symptoms in 12-14 hours, then venous thrombectomy is indicated.

Treatment by enzymatic means and by activation of the fibrinolytic system of the body offers many advantages. After a flurry of interest and popularity a number of years ago, followed by a period of apathy, these substances are once again gaining a rightful place in the treatment of venous disease. They are physiologic and actually restore patency and minimize the long-term sequelae usually seen in the postphlebitic extremity. The agent most commonly used at the present time is streptokinase. It has the advantage of having minimal side effects as compared to the previous preparations. However, these preparations are not suited at the present time for use in the pregnant patient or the postpartum patient with large areas of raw uterine surface, a recent episiotomy, or caesarean incision. Thus they are not utilized at this time in the gravid or postpartum female.

DISSEMINATED INTRAVENOUS THROMBOSIS

Disseminated intravenous thrombosis (DIC) is an unusual but troublesome problem in the obstetrical patient. In this syndrome there is a loss of balance between the body mechanisms for protection of the organism by producing clots and the lysis of activated coagulation products to maintain vascular integrity. (5) There are changes in consumption of platelets, and fibrinogen levels, and other coagulation factors are altered. Hardaway (10) states that there should be two conditions present for DIC to occur: (1) impairment of blood flow and (2) release of thromboplastic substances into the blood circulation. The stasis of flow may not be readily apparent, but the microvascular thrombosis from DIC impedes the flow and perpetuates the process. In the obstetrical patient, the underlying cause may be abruptio placenta, amniotic fluid embolism, the dead fetus syndrome, septic abortion, eclampsia, or the fatty liver of pregnancy.

Most often the phenomenon is manifested by abnormal bleeding, but in some cases the manifestation may be extensive and progressive thrombosis. It should be particularly suspect in a patient who has been hypotensive, particularly with one of the aforementioned clinical entities, who then develops abnormal bleeding.

To establish the diagnosis(5) a battery consisting of prothrombin time, platelet count, and fibrinogen levels provides a rapid and readily available screening profile. If all three are positive, the diagnosis is fairly firm. If there is still some doubt, then this can be expanded to prothrombin time, activated partial thromboplastin time, thrombin time, platelet count, fibrinogen levels, Factors V and VIII activity, tests for fibrin split products, and protamine sulfate paracoagulation. Depression of the platelet count, fibrinogen levels, Factors V and VII activity with prolongation of the prothrombin, partial thromboplastin and thrombin times, with elevation of the fibrin split products firmly secure the diagnosis. The protamine sulfate paracoagulation indicates circulating fibrin monomers and, when positive, is highly confirmative of DIC when the other factors are altered as above. (12)

Treatment includes (1) removing the underlying cause if feasible as, in the dead fetus syndrome, abruptio placenta or septic abortion, and (2) treating the other entities, eclampsia, fatty liver, and amniotic fluid embolism, and supportive measures to reverse acidosis and improve cardiac output, and general organ perfusion. Specific therapy for DIC consists of platelets, fresh frozen plasma, and anticoagulation of the patient with heparin by continuous infusion while monitoring the level by activated partial thromboplastin time (PTT). Usually the patient is begun on 800 units an hour, and PTT levels are done at six-hour intervals until the patient is stabilized at two to three times the control. This level is maintained from five to seven days until the abnormal bleeding or thrombosis is controlled and the hematologic values have been established. (See Table 7-1.)

Table 7-1

	Superficial Thrombophlebitis	Deep Venous Thrombosis (DVT)	Phlegmasia Alba Dolens	Phlegmasia Cerulea Dolens
Symptoms				
Onset	Varies	Insidious	Sudden	Slow
Pain	Minimal	Modest, maybe absent	Severe	Progressive
Findings				
Edema	0	+	+	+
Skin	Erythema	Normal	Pallid	Cyanotic
Motion	+	+	+	+
Pulses	+	+	May be decreased	Absent, late
Tenderness	Superficial, minimal	Deep + cuff test*	Deep + cuff test*	Deep + cuff test*
Venous distension	Absent to locally indurated	Significant when present	0	+ May be masked by edema
Relation to emboli	0	Major source	Rare	Same as DVT
Pathology	Superficial veins	Deep veins, pelvis + leg	Iliofemoral Suprainguinal Varies	Total deep system - Infrainguinal +
IPG + doppler	0	+		
Prognosis	Good	Related to further complications	Good if early treatment	Possible gangrene
Treatment	Local heat Support Aspirin	Local heat Elevation Bedrest Anticoagulant	Bedrest Anticoagulant Sympathetic Blockade Possible thrombectomy	Bedrest Elevation Local heat Early thrombectomy

*Cuff test: Intolerance to calf pressure by sphygmomanometer.

The mortality and morbidity of DIC can be severe. Collins et al. (5) in 1977 reported a 62% mortality in their series. Suspicion in the gravid patient, who has had one of the complications previously mentioned and who develops abnormal bleeding or a thrombotic process, should lead to prompt screening for DIC. Early diagnosis and early treatment will greatly improve the salvage rate in these patients.

PULMONARY EMBOLISM

Pulmonary embolism is not seen as a common problem in pregnancy but, as in the previously mentioned studies, presents with significant incidence and mortality. However, when it does occur, it presents a prolix of problems in regard to both diagnosis and treatment further convoluted by the presence of the fetus. Because of the anatomic and physiologic changes of pregnancy, the classical signs of chest pain, pleuritic pain, changes in respiration, and even peripheral edema may be masked, altered, or obscured. The patient usually has had some degree of chest discomfort or dyspnea. However, especially in the latter stages of pregnancy, with elevation of the diaphragm and alterations in respiration, these often are not present in a typical fashion. When tachycardia or hypotension are present, other causes secondary to pregnancy must be evaluated and ruled out. However, when the patient presents with chest pain, tachypnea, tachycardia, and dyspnea and there is no evidence of an obstetrical basis, then pulmonary embolization is the most suspect diagnosis.

Physical examination of the chest in the second and third trimesters may be compromised in regard to pleural rub or changes in aeration. The findings in the lower extremities also may be equivocal because of edema and venous hypertension of pregnancy. If the patient has an established diagnosis of deep venous thrombosis, the problem is less complicated and one can proceed to evaluation in the clinical or radiologic laboratory. Otherwise the noninvasive laboratory with doppler venous examination and venous plethysmography remains the mainstay in ruling upon the presence of a possible source of embolus in the lower extremities.

Clinical laboratory survey indicating a decrease in the arterial oxygen(12) PCO_2 with an increase in the pH is helpful in the diagnosis. A PCO_2 of less than 80 mm mercury was reported by Fairbairn et al. in a series of 36 patients.

In the electrocardiographic laboratory, some additional information may be obtained that will be helpful in the diagnosis. Quite often tachycardia, arrhythmia, depression of the ST

segments, and inversion of the T waves are additive information
of value in the workup.

Enzymatic changes were delineated by Walker et al., (12)
and there was a triad described in which there was an elevation
of the serum lactic acid dehydrogenase (LDH), hyperbilirubinemia (serum bilirubin elevated), and a normal serum glutamic-
oxalacetic transaminase. These are significant in the diagnosis
of pulmonary embolism or, if there is an absence of other diseases to account for an elevation of LDH, renal, hepatic, muscular, or neoplastic disease.

The final confirmation remains in the radiologic suite. Chest
roentgenology in pulmonary embolism without infarction may not
be of great value, especially if the embolus is small. However,
there may be elevation of the diaphragm on the affected side,
atelectasis, or unilateral effusion. If the embolus is large or
if there are multiple emboli present, changes can occur in the
pulmonary hilar shadows, and there may be areas of increased
density in the peripheral pulmonary fields. Perfusion and ventilation scanning remain, next to angiography, the most reliable
diagnostic tools radiologically. Perfusion scanning is carried
out by the infusion of macroaggregates of albumin tagged with
radioactive technetium. This substance accumulates in propor-
tion to the blood flow in the area. In pulmonary embolism there
is a decrease in these areas of flow or "cold" areas. To increase
the specificity, ventilation scanning with radioactive xenon can
be utilized. Comparison of the two, with the addition of a chest
x-ray, has a yield of 70-80% accuracy. In the patient with pulmonary embolization the ventilation scan reveals normal ventilation. However, in the patient with pneumonia, carcinoma, obstructive lung disease, or parenchymal changes these areas are
abnormal.

The use of radioactive isotopes(15) in the pregnant female
reveal a widespread range of opinions and practices. A significant number of researchers feel that any studies are contraindicated. Two reports from the United States Council on Radiation Protection and Measurement (NCRP) state the considerations offsetting radiation from medical radiation exposure to be
as follows:

1. "The medical welfare of both the expectant mother
    and the unborn child may be jeopardized if the indi-
    cated radiation procedures are not carried out."

2. "Recommends special care in selection of patients
    in certain cases of diagnostic radiology and nuclear
    medicine procedures."

In our institution, once the patient is aware of the hazards of perfusion and ventilation scanning, the procedure is carried out if agreeable to the patient and family. If possible, we attempt to avoid the first 14 weeks to minimize the tetrogenic effects. Most radiologists and nuclear medicine specialists feel the risk is tolerable when balanced against the information and implication of a lack of such knowledge.

Once the diagnosis has been established, the patient is treated by supportive measures for cardiac and pulmonary problems and anticoagulation by heparin in the same manner as the patient with DVT. Thus far we have not resorted to caval interruption or insertion of the intracaval prosthesis. In general, in the later stages of pregnancy, radiation hazards, the gravid uterus, and technical problems make these procedures not feasible. It is conceivable, in the patient at term who has not responded to the medical measures and who is having continued pulmonary emboli, that a combination of caesarean section and caval ligation would be feasible.

In the postpartum patient therapy is begun with heparin, bedrest, and supportive measures. However, if the patient has recurrence while on adequate anticoagulation of a pulmonary embolus, then caval plication or clipping of the vena cava with ligation of the left ovarian vein is utilized. Because of the venous dilatation in the recently gravid pelvis and the fact that the left ovarian vein enters the left renal vein separately, ligation is necessary.

Alternative treatment by the Mobin-Uddin umbrella or a Greenfield filter can be utilized. It has the advantage of local anesthesia and the absence of extensive surgical dissection. These prostheses, however, do have problems with error in placement. Because it is a semiblind procedure, local caval damage occurs on occasion and sometimes migration occurs to more proximal or distal portions of the circulation.

In the patient with pelvic abscess, infected abortion, or missed abortion, who has a septic embolus, direct and immediate ligation of the inferior vena cava with the initial episode is indicated because of the possibility of continued seeding and pulmonary abscess secondary to infected emboli.

There are a few miscellaneous conditions that remain: specifically, the patient with venous ulceration. These patients are treated by local cleansing with Betadine (providine iodine) three to four times daily and periodic irrigation during the day with peroxide. If the patient is hospitalized, such irrigation and debridement can be mechanically improved by using an apparatus consisting of an atomizer and oxygen under a mild degree of pressure for the irrigation source of the peroxide. The use of

Debrisan (dextranomer) powder and local scrupulous care of the granulation tissue often results in spontaneous healing. Wet to dry soaks additionally may be utilized to promote healthy granulation tissue. Some benefit may be gained by the use of a whirlpool. Periodic elevation during the day and external support by pressure gradient knee-length or waist-high garments are of great value.

It is a rare occasion for these patients to require skin grafting or excision. Such procedures, if possible, should wait until after delivery. Though bleeding from ulcerations or small spider nevi are rare complications, they do occur. Once again, these are managed by firm external support and elevation, but infrequently require surgical intervention for suture of the bleeding vessel.

The venous system is subjected to much stress as a result of the burden of pregnancy, but careful evaluation and an understanding of the anatomical and physiological reflections of this stage can guide one through these problems.

REFERENCES

1. Aaro, KA, and Juergens, JD. Thrombophlebitis and pulmonary embolism as complications of pregnancy, Med. Clin. N. Am., 58:829, 1974.

2. Aaro, KA, and Juergens, JL. Thrombophlebitis associated with pregnancy. Am. J. Obstet. Gynecol. 109:1128, 1971.

3. Alexander, P, Meyers, L, Kenny, J, Goldstein, R, Gurewich, V, and Grimspoon, L. Blood coagulation in pregnancy. N. Eng. J. Med., 254:358-363, 1956.

4. Cegelski, FC, DeWeese, JA, and Lurd, CJ. Deep iliofemoral venous thrombosis during pregnancy, Am. J. Obstet. Gynecol., 89:510, 1964.

5. Collins, GJ, Rich, NM, Scialla, S, Andersen, CA, and McDonald, PT. Pitfall in peripheral vascular surgery: Disseminated intravascular coagulation, Am. J. Surg., 134:375, 1977.

6. Coon, WW, Willis, PW, and Kellar, JB. Venous thromboembolism and other venous disease in the Tecumseh Community Health Study. Circulation, 48:839, 1973.

7. Dodd, H, and Cockett, FB. The Pathology and Surgery of the Veins of the Lower Limb. Edinburgh and London, E. & S. Livington, 1956.

8. Finnerty, JJ, and MacKay, BR. Antepartum thrombophlebitis and pulmonary embolism, Obstet. Gynecol., 19:405, 1962.

9. Friend, JR, and Kakkar, VV. Deep venous thrombosis in obstetric and gynecological patients. In Venous Thromboembolism, Madden, JL, and Hume, M, (Eds.). New York, Appleton-Century-Crofts, pp. 1-32, 1976.

10. Hardaway, RM. Disseminated intravascular coagulation as a possible cause of acute respiratory distress. Surg. Gynec. Obst., 137:419, 1973.

11. Hytten, FE, and Leitch, I. The Physiology of Human Pregnancy. Oxford, Blackwell Scientific Publications, 1964.

12. Juergens, JL, Spitell, Jr., JA, and Fairbairn, II, JF. Peripheral Vascular Disease. Philadelphia, London, Toronto, W.B. Saunders Co., pp. 768-769, 1980.

13. Marianus Sanctus Barolitanus. In Chirurgia: de Chirurgia Sciptorus Optinni. Zurich, Gessner, 1555.

14. McCausland, AM, Hyman, C, Winsor, T, and Fratter, AD. Venous distensibility during pregnancy. Am. J. Obstet. Gynecol., 77:1038, 1959.

15. Mole, RH. Radiation effects on prenatal development and their radiological significance, Br. J. Radiol., 52:614, 1979.

16. Moseley, P, and Kerstein, MD. Pregnancy and thrombophlebitis, Surg. Gynec. Obstet., 150:594, 1980.

17. Rose, DJ, Bader, ME, Bader, RA, and Braunwald, E. Catheterization studies of cardiac hemodynamics in normal pregnant women. Am. J. Obstet. 72:233, 1956.

18. Villasanta, V. Thromboembolic disease complicating pregnancy, Am. J. Obstet. Gynecol., 93:142, 1954.

19. Walters, WAW, and Lim, YL. Changes in the maternal cardiovascular system during human pregnancy. _Surg. Gynec. Obstet._ , 135:765, 1970.

20. White, PW, Sadd, JR, and Nensel, RE. Thrombotic complications of heparin therapy. _Am. J. Surg._ , 190:5, 1979.

Chapter 8

BREAST DISEASES DURING PREGNANCY

Robert T. Tidrick, M.D.

INTRODUCTION

The physician caring for the pregnant patient may encounter
evidence of a current breast lesion or may be informed of a
past history of benign or malignant disease. Fortunately, most
breast cancers occur beyond the childbearing years. There are,
however, a large number of benign breast disorders which occur
during pregnancy and must be clarified in terms of their diagnosis and need for treatment. It must be emphasized that the
initial visit of the pregnant patient should include careful in-
quiry about previous breast problems, assessment of risk factors in relation to breast cancer, and a careful examination of
the breasts. If there have been previous diagnostic measures
directed at her breasts, such as radiographic examinations or
biopsies, the information derived from these tests must be evaluated. The earlier these matters can be clarified during pregnancy, the better in terms of ensuring an uneventful pregnancy
and achievement of successful management of the breast problem.

In considering the subject of breast cancer as it occurs during pregnancy or lactation, one must ask a series of questions
and explore each of these in a historical sense. What end results lead to the generally accepted pessimism regarding the
problem of breast cancer presenting during pregnancy? Are the
early survival statistics valid in comparison with those of today? Does the state of pregnancy necessarily impose grave
prognosis in the patient who presents with cancer of the breast?
If survival chances are reduced, what factors are responsible,
at least potentially, for this lessened prognosis? Are these due
principally to changes in the hormonal milieu and decline in the
immune competence of such patients? Does treatment during

pregnancy carry with it high risk to the developing fetus? Do operations directed against the cancer during the latter half of pregnancy gravely affect long-term survival? Does the delay of definitive treatment until after delivery constitute high risk of impaired survival for those encountered late in the second half of pregnancy? Does lactation and nursing the infant following previous treatment of breast cancer tend to "light-up" or activate dormant disease? Does subsequent pregnancy in the patient who has had a previously treated breast cancer decrease the chances of survival? If a patient desires to have a subsequent child or children, what should be the optimum interval advised following the treatment of the cancer before an ensuing pregnancy is commenced? What is the risk of developing a second cancer in the remaining breast? What morphological characteristics of the original neoplasm might give a clue to increased risk of a second primary carcinoma? What diagnostic measures may a physician employ during the course of pregnancy to rule in or rule out the presence of a malignant lesion? What measures may be taken to render the diagnostic measures of maximum safety to the mother and fetus? Is interruption of pregnancy due to the presence of malignant breast tumor justified and, if so, under what conditions might this possibility be entertained? Would prophylactic oophorectomy or radiation sterilization following delivery lessen the chances of recurrent or metastatic disease and increase survival?

These are the questions which will be attended to in the following pages and which constitute those parts of a complex problem which the family physician, the obstetrician, and the surgeon may be confronted. The common benign conditions will first be discussed and suggestions made regarding their diagnosis and possible treatment.

COMMON BENIGN CONDITIONS

Benign Diseases Which May Need Consideration During Pregnancy

Chronic cystic mastitis

Fat necrosis

Plasma cell mastitis

Chronic ductal ectasia

Galactocele

Chronic suppurative mastitis, including ductal fistula

Papilloma and papillomatosis

Adenoma of nipple

Fibroadenoma

Chronic Cystic Mastitis

Fibrocystic disease is a catchall term also referred to as
chronic cystic mastitis. It has broad application in clinical
diagnosis. It appears basically as a disturbed relationship of
the breast parenchyma through hormonal influences and possibly
through other factors which may contribute to disturbances in
ductal and acinar epithelium and stroma. It is applied to those
women with nodular breasts who may have premenstrual pain
and tenderness. The disease is usually bilateral. On palpation,
such breasts tend to be dense and multinodular. Mammographic
or xeroradiographic examination usually shows increased fibrosis, ductal prominence, and, in some instances, associated
cysts. Small cysts or microcysts predominate, but in some
instances there may be the appearance of large cysts which
comprise the so-called "blue domed" cysts. The cysts are usually lined by a single layer of epithelium and, in themselves,
are rarely related to any malignant change. Microscopic examination usually demonstrates various degrees of ductal hyperplasia. The extent of this hyperplasia and its cellular appearance may be a guide in determining the degree of risk which may
exist in terms of the development of breast cancer. This may
present as multilayering of ductal epithelium or as plugging of
the collecting or terminal ducts. One may find areas of apocrine
metaplasia. This form usually assumes a papillary pattern.
There are varying degrees of parenchymal disruption due to
periductal and perilobular hyperplasia of connective tissue.
This fibrosis may become a predominant part of the picture.
The collagen may appear dense, hypocellular, and often hyalin-
ized. Distortion of the breast pattern is inevitable.

Clinical presentation of women with fibrocystic disease is
usually between the ages of 25 and 45; manifestations are uncommon after the menopause. The exact relationship of fibrocystic disease to the risk of cancer has long been a question
that even now has not been entirely resolved. The fact that there
exists some degree of increased risk appears evident, and this

is presumably due to the type and extent of ductal hyperplasia.
Biopsy is frequently necessary, with special concern in the
frozen section examination of the patient with sclerosing adeno-
sis. The differentiation of this entity from infiltrating ductal
carcinoma is often difficult and may even create problems with
fixed tissue section interpretation. The major problem in management of the patient with florid fibrocystic disease is in differ-
entiating it from malignancy through physical examination and
radiographic means. The conditions do not require treatment
during pregnancy, but do require consideration in terms of differential diagnosis. As pregnancy progresses, the physical
findings tend to be masked as gestational hyperplasia progresses.

Fat Necrosis

This is most frequently seen in the obese patient with pendulous breasts. It may occur, perhaps in one-half of the instances,
from known antecedent trauma and is occasionally seen after
breast biopsy. In rare instances, it has been seen in conjunction
with Weber-Christian disease. The firmness of the mass and
changes in overlying skin may cause it to be confused with carcinoma. (1) Although it can occur during pregnancy, it is more
likely to be seen in those beyond childbearing years.

Plasma Cell Mastitis

This entity unmistakably overlaps with fat necrosis. The
lesion is characterized by an area of dense fibrosis heavily infiltrated with chronic inflammatory cells in which plasma cells
may predominate. There may be areas of fat necrosis. As in
classic fat necrosis, the changes in overlying skin, the firmness of the involved mass, and even occasionally retraction of
the nipple may cause great difficulty in differentiation from carcinoma and can only be ascertained by appropriate biopsy. (2)

Ductal Ectasia

These ductal changes are predominantly involutional in origin.
The principle or collecting ducts fill with desquamated epithelial
debris, dilate, and create periductal fibrosis. They may be associated with a chronic thick and nonbloody nipple discharge.
Ductal ectasia may be present as a part of the panorama in fibrocystic disease. The physical findings may also simulate carcinoma, especially in those lesions of central location. There
are significant interrelationships among these clinical and
pathological entities, and frequent use of biopsy is needed in
their clarification.

Galactocele and Galactorrhea

Galactocele may present as a persistent cystic mass in the parous woman. It may or may not demonstrate ductal communication to produce the appearance of a milky, ductal discharge. Its nature frequently may be determined by aspiration, which sometimes suffices to be curative. Problems in differential diagnosis may exist if the mass is deep, thick-walled, or surrounded by considerable reaction. Persistent lactiferous drainage may persist for a time if it is incompletely emptied.

Persistent galactorrhea may appear in a nonpregnant woman and should be investigated by obtaining prolactin levels. Mild prolactin elevation may occur when the patient is taking certain forms of birth control medication, and, in these cases, discontinuation of the hormones may be curative. If the prolactin elevation is significantly high, additional investigation is needed to rule out the presence of a prolactin-secreting adenoma of the pituitary.

Chronic Suppurative Mastitis, Including Ductal Fistula

Acute suppurative mastitis associated with lactation may present as a relatively superficial subareolar mass, as a deeper interlobar mass with the principle collection within the depths of the breast parenchyma, or, in more severe instances, as a retro- or submammary abscess. Persistent suppurative mastitis may occur from incomplete drainage of a deep abscess; in the process, there may be progression to that of a chronic phlegmon in the subacute or chronic form.

The most common form encountered is seen in the nonlactating woman, often associated with persistent ductal fistula. In these cases there is repeated presentation of infection, usually at the periphery of the areola. One is likely to find the association of a congenitally fissured nipple. The crevice in the nipple serves as a site of low-grade infection, which presumably involves the underlying lactiferous sinus or sinuses, and then presents in the areola or at its border as the process spreads beyond the involved duct or ducts. Elective correction of the fistulation is to be encouraged. When the process continues into pregnancy, it contraindicates nursing the infant.

Ductal Papilloma or Papillomatosis

The principal presenting sign of a ductal papilloma is frankly bloody discharge from a nipple orifice. This is most likely to be apparent in the patient who is in her thirties or forties.

These lesions may grow to sufficient size to be palpated and cause ductal dilatation and stasis. One must differentiate between intraductal papilloma and diffuse or multiple papillomatosis of the ducts. The latter is characterized by bloody discharge or ductal fluid, giving a positive test for occult blood. The discharge comes from multiple-duct orifices and may present bilaterally. Frozen section examination of ductal papilloma may be difficult and has occasionally led to erroneous diagnosis of cancer and overtreatment. (3) Localization of the involved segment with local wedge resection of the involved duct and immediate adjoining parenchyma is usually sufficient. The localization is easy if there is a palpable mass. Mammography, xeroradiography, or sonography may be helpful in localization. The traditional method of determining which radial segment produces expression of the bloody discharge by finger pressure may not always be sufficient. Occasionally, catherization of the involved nipple orifice, with a fine, plastic catheter, and injection of a dye may be quite helpful in identifying the involved segment when appropriate exposure of the involved quadrant is done. Contrast radiographic methods have been reported. (4)

Diffuse papillomatosis presents a much more difficult problem in management. Its diffuseness and the degree of the accompanying hyperplasia should be evaluated by appropriate bilateral biopsies. One must be cognizant that bloody nipple discharge, whether in the single or multiple orifice, is an indication for the immediate institution of appropriate diagnostic measures. These start with obtaining adequate preparations for cytology interpretation. The results cannot be given the same credence as biopsy information.

Adenoma of the Nipple

The diagnosis is ordinarily easily made and excision is a simple matter. Occasionally, in those of long-standing and bulky size, superficial ulceration may occur and lead to confusion as to whether Paget's disease exists. Appropriate microscopic examination may be necessary to differentiate.

Fibroadenoma

Peak age occurs between 18 and 35. A number of observers have seen an apparent racial difference, noting a subset of fibroadenomas that appear at an earlier age in puberty in young black females and which appear to grow rapidly and often reach a bulky size. Increase in the size of fibroadenoma has been reported during pregnancy. They are usually single but may present as multiple lesions. The physical findings are usually typical: well demarcated, moveable, firm, and, if reasonably superficial, give the impression of having a smooth outline. They are ordinarily oval or discoid but may be multilobulated. In older women, one may find such a lesion to have become calcified or, in some instances, even ossified and exceedingly hard. Microscopically, they are divided into two main types – the more common intracanalicular form, in which the connective tissue overgrowth is so prominent as to compress the ductal structures into invaginated slits, and the less common pericanalicular form, which shows much more abundant ductal proliferation and may demonstrate more cellularity of the fibrous stroma. The ductal distortion characteristic of the former type is absent. There is some overlap of the two forms. It is the pericanalicular type which is more likely to be seen in the young pubertal patient.

Cystosarcoma phyllodes represents a sarcomatous form of fibrous tissue tumor which bears a number of relationships to fibroadenoma. In some fibroadenomas characterized by progressive growth, the term "giant fibroadenoma" is applied. Drawing the line between "giant fibroadenoma" and cystosarcoma is difficult. The microscopic interpretation hinges largely on the evidence of stromal changes indicative of progressive and rapid growth. Cystosarcoma phyllodes metastasize only rarely and then by hematogenous means. There have been a few rare reports of the combination of stromal malignancy (that is, cystosarcoma phyllodes) and accompanying or associated epithelial malignancy. (5) If there is a history of rapid growth of a fibroadenoma encountered early in pregnancy, it should be removed. Those of relatively small size and with a record of sluggish growth may be followed through the pregnancy if there is reasonable assurance of the firmness of the diagnosis.

CANCER OF THE BREAST

The human breast exhibits considerable variation in its structure during the stages of long life. The infantile or prepubertal breast shows but rudimentary duct structures and is seldom the source of any clinical concern. In adolescence, there is active proliferation with the development of ductal and lobular structures. These culminate in the adult characteristics of the breast during the reproductive span of life. Lesions of the breast coming to clinical attention in the pubertal period are usually fibroadenomata. During the span of the reproductive period, the breast is the site of constant change owing to the seesaw of hormonal activity. The cyclic changes synchronized with the menstrual cycle may be interrupted from time to time by the major proliferative stimuli of pregnancy and lactation.

The postmenopausal breast is the site of atrophic or senescent changes. These may be delayed or interrupted by hormonal stimulation, exogenous administration, or an unnatural occurrence, as in the production of estrogen by the ovary or from adrenal source.

Our principal concern is with that aspect of mammary cancer in which there is coincidence with, or, at least, appearance during, pregnancy. The significant changes which occur in the breast during pregnancy must be considered from two standpoints: first, how these profound cellular and hormonal changes, increase in vascularity, and alterations in immune competence may in themselves accelerate breast cancer; and second, to what extent these changes interfere with the appropriate recognition of the neoplasm or cause treatment to be postponed or diminished in extent. The problems, of course, involve not only the mother and the patient, but also the fetus.

The evolution of the surgical treatment of cancer of the breast occurred slowly during the nineteenth century. Credit is given to William S. Halsted(6) and Willy Meyer(7) for introducing the radical mastectomy in the last decade of the nineteenth century. The basis of their extension of the area of ablation, to include regional lymph nodes, was founded on the belief or assumption that mammary cancer was, for a considerable part of its natural history, a local, and then a regional, disease Occurring from time to time were brief references to the occurrence of pregnancy or lactation coincident with cancer of the breast, and there were gloomy statements indicating a pessimistic, if not hopeless, view. These views continued to dominate surgical attitudes until the past two decades, during which there has been not only a change in the pessimistic view about the influences of pregnancy and lactation, but also profound expansion of our concepts concerning the impact biological influences have on the complex problem of breast cancer.

Credit is rightfully assigned to Beatson(8), in Edinburgh, for introducing the role of hormonal influence in the behavior of breast cancer. He observed the delay in progress of metastatic mammary cancer following oophorectomy. Clinical trials were by the signal work of Huggins(9) in relation to prostatic and breast cancer, with the availability of increasingly purified and available estrogens and androgens.

The laboratory methods which became available in the middle decades of this century have made it possible to study the changes in the hormonal milieu occurring in pregnancy and lactation. There is a striking rise in estrogen levels during pregnancy (up to a 300-fold increase). Of the three estrogen components, the most significant elevation is that of estriol, followed by estrone, and then by estradiol. Circulating adrenocortical steroid levels are increased 2- to 3-fold. During lactation, there are elevated levels of prolactin. Whether or not this has a deleterious effect on breast cancers in the human is not clear, although there is evidence that it is deleterious in mouse and rat models. (10, 11)

There has been accelerated interest in the relationship of humoral and cellular immunity in cancer, partly as a product of the intensive studies in transplant biology and modern oncology. There is considerable evidence that immunity is impaired during pregnancy. Strelkuskas(12), in 1975, reported depression of circulating T- and B-lymphocytes during pregnancy, and others have reported depressed cellular immune response. Evidence from studies of hormonal changes and diminution in immune competence give credence to some of the pessimism which has characterized the attitude toward treatment and prognosis. Certainly it appears logical that the increased vascularity and presumed increased lymphatic flow, which progresses throughout pregnancy, would accelerate the spread to metastatic sites by both hematogenous and lymphatic routes.

Do survival statistics confirm these earlier views? Has such pessimism, based on earlier random observations, continued to influence early recognition and appropriate therapy for the gravid woman with cancer of the breast? Most surgeons and obstetricians are not likely to have very extensive personal experiences. In America and the cold-climate countries of Western Europe, almost three-quarters of breast cancers appear after the reproductive period has entirely ceased.

In reviewing 45,881 cases from various reports, White(13), in 1955, found 2.8% coincident with or in women who had had a recent pregnancy. In 1973, Applewhite(14) found, in 655 women of childbearing age or under 45 years, 7.3% pregnant or lactating. However, Treves and Holleb(15), reviewing a younger group, found that in 549 patients less than 35 years of age, 14% had concurrent cancer. In America, Donegan(16) has estimated that only 17% of breast cancer occurs in the childbearing years.

Survival studies in the past two decades have indicated some optimism and give support to a more aggressive view toward management. While Cheek(17), in 1953, found that in a survey of 47 authorities not more than 5.3% survived five years, Peters and colleagues(18, 19) have, in reports (1965, 1968), lent support to a view with a less ominous tone. Peters, in studying 187 patients, found a deficit in survival of 10-15% at five years. These patients were carefully matched by age and stage with those who were not pregnant. Applewhite(14), in 1973, found 15% survived at 10 years. It would appear from the evidence that if one matches age, stage of disease, type of neoplasm, and kind and extent of treatment with the nonpregnant woman, survival is not substantially worse.

As a generalization, there is probably some increment of delay in establishing a diagnosis when the pregnant patient presents with a mass in the breast, and engorgement of the breasts makes delineation of a mass difficult. The risk of casual consideration of a dominant mass in the pregnant patient expands as the pregnancy progresses. Emphasis should be placed on having a very careful examination at the first prenatal visit. It should be stressed that this examination should include careful inspection in adequate light, with the patient seated, and include viewing the breasts from several angles. This should be done with the patient's arm first at repose, then abducted, and finally extended overhead with tensing of the pectoral muscles. In examining a woman with pendulous breasts, the examination should include forward bending to exclude tethering of a deep mass to the underlying pectoral fascia. Palpation of the breast while the patient is recumbent on the examining table should be done first with one shoulder, and then the other, elevated on a pillow or pad so that the breast is flattened as much as possible on the chest wall. If a mass is located or suspected from this palpation, examination should include the additional steps of moistening the skin with a water-soluble lubricant and evaluating the mass with light, circular finger movements.

In few other clinical situations is a "wait and see" plan less applicable. Assuming that a dominant mass is found in the first prenatal examination, its nature should be investigated at that time. If the physical characteristics suggest that it is a cyst, aspiration is applicable. A small amount of appropriate, local anesthetic is injected in the overlying skin and the mass is penetrated with a obturated #22-gage, short, beveled needle. The obturator is removed and suction applied. If fluid is obtained and cytology laboratory facilities are close at hand, the syringe containing fluid should be delivered so that centrifugation and study of the sediment can be done. If these facilities are not available, appropriate glass-slide smears may be made and immediate fixation done. If fluid is obtained and the impression of a cyst confirmed, one must ascertain that the mass is gone. If the mass being aspirated appears to be solid, strong suction is applied and then released before the needle is withdrawn. The syringe is uncoupled from the needle, the plunger is drawn back to introduce air, and the cellular contents of the needle are forcefully blown on a slide. Immediate fixation is mandatory. The yield in finding tumor cells in aspirated cyst fluid is quite low. The solid mass aspirate may yield helpful information, but negative findings must not deter the clinician from early additional diagnostic measures including biopsy.

X-ray film mammography or xeroradiography can be performed during pregnancy. Because of pregnancy hyperplasia, vascular engorgement, and attendant increase in density, there are difficulties in interpretation. There is reluctance on the part of patients and physicians alike to employ radiation sources of diagnosis during pregnancy. However, the risks from such examinations of the breast are low if appropriate precautions are taken. The usual practice is simply to screen the remainder of the body with two of the protective aprons employed by radiologists. With the progressive improvement in ultrasonic scanning equipment, there being at least three such devices designed exclusively for breast examination, there exists a modality that can distinguish with good accuracy cystic from solid masses and is especially helpful in deep-seated lesions. The use of the dedicated, automated breast scanner represents a significant advance over the use of hand-held scanning equipment — the delineation of masses is not as sharp as with mammography or xeroradiography, microcalcific shadows are not seen, there is no ionizing radiation involved, and many views from diverse angles can be obtained.

Biopsy is the bedrock upon which a logical course of action can be established. Reluctance to perform biopsy during pregnancy should be abandoned. Much of this reluctance is based on the fear of adverse effects on the pregnancy. It is mandatory that there be close cooperation between the patient's physician caring for the pregnancy and the surgeon who is to perform the biopsy. The use of local anesthesia, except for superficial and small masses, is not recommended. Its use in deep-seated masses can be frustrating and unsatisfactory. Modern general anesthesia and skills render the risk to mother and fetus negligible.

What if the biopsy is positive? The treatment of the cancer is of highest priority. One may speculate that some of the poor survival reported in earlier years was in part due to long postponement of therapy until after completion of the pregnancy. The other aspect of this decreased survival probably was due to more patients appearing with advanced disease when first detected during the pregnancy.

Several decades ago, the risk of fetal loss was high when operation was performed during pregnancy. In 1937, Harrington(20) reported 36% risk of fetal loss in pregnant patients operated upon at the Mayo Clinic in 1910-1933. In contrast, Byrd(21), in 1962, reported on 86 patients subject to operation during pregnancy with only one spontaneous abortion in the group. He expressed his view succinctly when answering the question of whether the pregnancy should be terminated when cancer of the breast is diagnosed: his answer was "terminate the cancer, not the pregnancy." It would appear that, as a generalization, this is a sound principle. The indications for termination would appear to be few and include those with advanced cancer and patently obvious incurability, with very limited life expectancy. It is obvious that radiation therapy, use of chemotherapeutic drugs, or hormonal alteration cannot be effected during pregnancy lest there be grave risk to the fetus. There is a very small group of mammary cancer patients who present with undifferentiated or so-called inflammatory carcinoma. These present a dismal and almost uniformly fatal prognosis, although some may respond to therapy. (22) Surgical treatment at any stage of the disease is often considered futile, and, if radiation therapy or chemotherapy are to be employed, they obviously cannot be used during the intrauterine life of the fetus. Should a very early pregnancy be terminated because of greater risk of damage to the developing embryo? One cannot find evidence to substantiate the view that the presence of the cancer per se creates hazard in terms of causing birth defects.

What should be our attitude based upon the stage of pregnancy? Certainly treatment should start promptly if the lesion is discovered in the first half of the pregnancy. It would appear that postponement of treatment in the second trimester carries too long a delay and is against the best interest of the mother. If discovery of the malignant lesion occurs during the third trimester, should there be postponement for a few weeks until delivery is accomplished? Or, should there be pressure to effect early premature labor and termination of pregnancy as soon as there is reasonable assurance of a viable infant? These questions having to do with possible early termination of pregnancy or accelerating the date of delivery are difficult and must be made with the informed participation of the patient and her family. It would appear that some degree of compromise is in the interest of both mother and fetus.

What surgical procedures should be performed in the pregnant patient with an established diagnosis of infiltrating ductal carcinoma? This type is the most commonly encountered, comprising about 75% of the total in most series. The logical procedure is to perform a satisfactory cancer operation, encompassing no more nor less than one would with a patient matched with the same age and stage who is not pregnant. If surgical treatment is planned, current practice would be to remove the breast with axillary node dissection, either employing the Auchincloss procedure(23) with preservation of both pectoral muscles, or the Patey(24) procedure with excision of the pectoralis minor muscle. Hemostasis during pregnancy is somewhat more complicated, but not unduly difficult.

In the third trimester consideration should be given to effect a compromise, briefly delay definitive treatment, and accelerate delivery. Having embarked on this course of compromise, it appears logical that one must take such measures to insure a high likelihood of survival of the infant if prematurity of several weeks is anticipated. This may include performance of amniocentesis to insure that there is adequate fetal lung development. It should also provide for delivery to take place under circumstances that can provide expert care for a premature infant. If there is substantial prematurity, say 35 to 36 weeks of gestation, it may not be possible to induce labor and caesarean section may become necessary. The question of performing oophorectomy at this time is occasionally raised. As a prophylactic measure in the woman who is free of evidence of disseminated disease, the answer is negative. It not only adds castration **sequelae to an already disturbed** situation, but it removes this possible modality of treatment from the armamentarium of the premenopausal woman in the event that there is subsequent evidence of dissemination and possible need for oophorectomy. Evidence that prophylactic oophorectomy may postpone the appearance of dissemination or extend life is lacking. (25, 26) Having compromised in both the timing of definitive treatment and in hastening delivery, there is no need for procrastination in proceding with treatment in the course of ten days to two weeks if the puerperium has been smooth. Lactation is promptly brought to a halt by hormonal means. Isotope skeletal scans should be performed and other measures deemed necessary to rule out the presence of disseminated disease prior to embarking on mastectomy or partial breast excision.

In any instance, the surgeon and the physician caring for the patient during her pregnancy must consider alternate forms of treatment and present the alternatives to the patient and her family. The alternative which is most applicable is to consider radiation therapy. This refers to wide excision of the primary lesion followed by radiation therapy. The employment of radiation therapy with removal of a limited portion of the breast, as an alternate treatment form, is widely practiced in patients with stage I or stage II carcinomas. In current use is the method of employing external beam therapy, using photons with an [6]MEV accelerator, with augmentation of the local area by interstitial treatment after completion of the external beam therapy to the breast and adjoining lymph node groups.

Whether axillary lymph node sampling or complete axillary dissection should be done at the time of local excision is perhaps controversial at this time. Correlation is low between the physical findings relative to the presence or absence of axillary metastasis and the status of the lymph nodes as demonstrated histologically. The information gained from the examination of the axillary lymph nodes is extremely helpful in appropriate staging. The presence or absence of axillary lymph node involvement is of vital importance in shaping the decisions to be made in relation to adjunctive therapy. In the event radiation therapy is selected as the principal treatment, complete removal of the axillary nodes lessens the need to heavily irradiate the area of the apex of the underlying lung.

The term "lumpectomy" is sometimes used to describe the local excision of the primary tumor. This term, by its implication, should be abandoned. The more elegant term "tylectomy" may be preferred. There should be wide excision of the tumor. Provision for estrogen and progesterone receptor assay on the tumor should be obtained. There is scant information pertaining to interpretation of such tumor cell assays during human pregnancy.

The procedures involved in radiation therapy have not stood the test of extended time of observation. A small number of patients have multifocal disease and local excision is inadequate. There are some complications of late radiation therapy, although these appear to be lessened with currently used methods. (27) In all instances, appropriate consultation should be obtained and options presented before embarking upon definitive therapy.

Histological types other than infiltrating ductal carcinoma or undifferentiated carcinoma may, if found, have some bearing on decisions in relation to treatment. The higher-than-usual incidence of bilaterality in lobular carcinoma is well documented and should direct early attention to the opposite breast. The presence of medullary or colloid carcinoma will not alter treatment plans. Low-grade papillary carcinoma, intraductal carcinoma, and lobular carcinoma in situ may not only provide some anguish for the pathologist confronted with the pregnancy hyperplasia in the same breast, but occasionally lead to a decision to postpone definitive therapy until after completion of the pregnancy. This is not recommended, but definitive diagnosis in some of these may be difficult.

There are clinical questions of some importance pertaining to lactation. Reference has been made earlier to the possible adverse effect of prolactin on growth of mammary neoplasms in rodents. Such a link has not been clearly demonstrated in the human. Nevertheless, one can hardly condone a view that, because of lack of such proof, such a relationship does not exist. If, during pregnancy, a tumor is found in the patient's breast which proves to be malignant on appropriate biopsy, and treatment is carried out during or shortly after completion of

the pregnancy, the assumption of nursing of the infant is not likely to occur and would be contraindicated. Not only would continued elevation of prolactin levels occur with the possible adverse
effects discussed, but adjuvant therapy, if indicated by the stage
and type of the cancer, would be out of the question while the infant is being nursed. The question of the possible role of mammary cancer viruses has been an intriguing one since Bittner(28)
reported, in 1936, his experiments with vertical transmission
of viruses in mice through the mother's milk. The possible
transmission of viruses in the milk of the nursing human mother,
in contrast to Bittner's mice, has never been proved in spite of
continued interest and experiments. The question of whether or
not any woman who, in the past, has had successful treatment of
breast cancer and a subsequent pregnancy, should be permitted
or encouraged to nurse the infant, has never been fully answered.

The young patient who has had one pregnancy coinciding with
mammary cancer may bring the question of a planned subsequent
pregnancy to her physician. Before a logical answer can be
given it is desirable to consider the stage and type of neoplasm
which was present. In the instance of the patient with proved
axillary lymph node metastasis, adjunctive therapy is usually
indicated. The prognosis for long-term survival is significantly
diminished. If the stage and tumor type indicate the need for
adjunctive therapy, this has high priority. The accumulating
evidence from use of multidrug chemotherapy indicates that, as
a measure employed in high-risk subjects, the free interval is
extended before appearance of dissemination occurs. Whether
duration of survival is lengthened is not clear. The patient
whose prognosis for long-term survival is very guarded because
of distant or recurrent disease should be very strongly discour-
aged from becoming pregnant. The child's probable early loss
of mother involves ethical and philosophical questions the patient and her family would have to consider. The presence of
intercurrent pregnancy would materially narrow options for
appropriate palliative treatment of metastatic disease. If the
patient is insistent upon having another child, it would seem
logical to consider an interval of three years, inasmuch as during this period recurrent or metastatic disease is most likely
to become manifest. Unfortunately, dissemination is frequently
present at the time the tumor is first recognized. While this
likelihood bears a strong relationship to stage, tumor size, and
histological type, there exists a sizable margin of uncertainty.
One uses as a guide those statistics based on the behavior of a
large number of such neoplasms. Romsdahl(29), in a follow-up
of 177 patients, found that there was recurrence of 29% in the
first year, 30% during the second year, and 13% during the third

year. An additional 20% showed recurrence between the fourth
and eleventh years. In other studies, it has been indicated that
the period in which dissemination is most likely to become evident lies within the first three years after treatment. Even in
the patient with favorable prognosis, that is, one in whom the
primary tumor is small and no lymph node metastasis is demonstrable, a similar waiting period is logical. The idea that pregnancy "lights up" dormant breast cancer has not been substantiated.

Any patient who has had a carcinoma in one breast is in con-
tinuing peril of developing one in the remaining breast. In overall
terms this is estimated by most to be at 1%/year. The need for
regular systematic screening for the remainder of the lifetime
is obvious. In a patient who has had a lobular carcinoma, the
chances of synchronous bilaterality is high (estimated to be 30%).
Minimum screening in those at continuous risk should consist
of careful instruction of the patient in monthly self-examination,
physician examination every six months, and x-ray mammography or xeroradiography every year. In the young patient, consideration should be given to subcutaneous mastectomy with use
of implant or other reconstruction measures. This should especially be given consideration if there has been postmastectomy
reconstruction on the side from which the original neoplasm was
removed. While subcutaneous mastectomy does not entirely remove the risk, it lessens the likelihood of contralateral neoplasm. The use of hormonal agents in effecting contraception
in those who have had mammary cancers is theoretically un-
desirable, although evidence to bolster this view is lacking.

SUMMARY

Benign diseases of the breast are more likely to be present
than malignant lesions. They constitute special problems in
the pregnant patient in differentiation from cancer. Determi-
nation of their nature, which may require special diagnostic
measures or treatment prior to completion of pregnancy, may
tax the skills of those attending the patient.

Carcinoma of the breast presenting during pregnancy requires
treatment which should not involve unnecessary delay, subopti-
mal methods, or unnecessary radicalism. The welfare of mother
and fetus must be considered, and such accommodation as has
to be made because of the pregnancy should not depart from accepted standards of cancer therapy. The results of therapy, if
compared to the nonpregnant patient when stage and type of disease are considered, do not justify the pessimism of former

times. The questions of subsequent childbearing and nursing are ones which confront those who counsel such patients.

REFERENCES

1. Adair, FE, and Munzer, JT. Fat necrosis of the female breast. Am. J. Surg., 74:117-128, 1947.

2. Adair, FE. Plasma cell mastitis: A lesion simulating mammary carcinoma. Arch. Surg., 26:735-749, 1933.

3. Kraus, FT, and Neubecker, RD. The differential diagnosis of papillary tumors of the breast. Cancer, 15:444-455, 1962.

4. Goes, JS, and Goes, JCS. Progress in clinical and biological research, Vol. 12. In Breast Cancer. New York: Alan R. Liss, Inc., 1977, pp. 151-282.

5. Gittleman, MA, and Horstmann, JP. Cystosarcoma phyllodes with concurrent infiltrating ductal carcinoma. Breast, 9:1, 15-17, Jan.-Mar. 1983.

6. Halstead, WS. The results of operations for the cure of cancer of the breast performed at the John Hopkins Hospital from June, 1889 to Jan., 1894. Ann. Surg., 20:497-555, 1894.

7. Meyer, W. An improved method of the radical operation for carcinoma of the breast. M. Rec., 46:746, 1894.

8. Beatson, GT. On the treatment of inoperable cases of carcinoma of the mamma: Suggestions for a new treatment with illustrative cases. Lancet, 2:104-107, 162-165, 1896.

9. Huggins, C. Endocrine substances in the treatment of cancers. JAMA, 14:750-754, 1949.

10. Stoll, BA. Secondary spread in breast cancer, Vol. 3. In New Aspects of Breast Cancer. New York: Wm. Heinemann Med. Books Ltd., 1977, p. 170.

11. Montague, ACW. Progress in clinical and biological research, Vol. 12. In Breast Cancer. New York: Alan R. Liss, Inc., 1977, pp. 155-163.

12. Strelkausas, AJ, Wilson, BE, and Dray, D, et al. Inversion of levels of human T and B cells in early pregnancy. Nature, 258:331, 1975.

13. White, TT. Prognosis of breast cancer for pregnant and nursing women: Analysis of 1,413 cases. Surg. Gynec. Obstet., 100:661-666, 1955.

14. Applewhite, RR, Smith, LR, and DiVicenti, F. Carcinoma of the breast associated with pregnancy and lactation. Ann. Surg., 39:101, 1973.

15. Treves, N, and Holleb, AI. A report of 549 cases of breast cancer in women 35 years of age or younger. Surg. Gynec. Obstet., 107:271-283, 1958.

16. Donagen, WL. Chapter 19. In Breast Cancer Management, Early and Late. Stoll, BA (Ed.). Wm. Heinemann Med. Books Ltd., distributed by Year Book Medical Publishers, 1977.

17. Cheek, JH. Survey of current options concerning carcinoma of the breast occurring during pregnancy. Arch. Surg., 66:664, 1953.

18. Peters, MB, and Meakin, JW. Vol. 1. In Progress in Clinical Cancer, Ariel, IM (Ed.). New York: Grune & Stratton, 1965, pp. 471-506.

19. Peters, MV. Effects of pregnancy in breast cancer. In Prognostic Factors in Breast Cancer, Forrest, ATM, and Kunkler, PB (Eds.). Edinboro: Livingstone, 1968, p. 383.

20. Harrington, SW. Carcinoma of the breast: Results of surgical treatment when the carcinoma occurred in the course of pregnancy or lactation and when pregnancy occurred subsequent to operation (1910-1933). Ann. Surg., 106:690-700, 1937.

21. Byrd, BS, Bayer, DS, Robertson, JC, and Stephenson, SA. Treatment of breast tumors associated with pregnancy and lactation. Ann. Surg., 155:940-947, 1962.

22. Pollak, EW, and Getzin, LC. Inflammatory carcinoma of the breast: Therapeutic approach followed by improved survival. Am. J. Surg., 136:722-725, Dec. 1978.

23. Auchincloss, H. Significance of location and number of axillary metastases in carcinoma of the breast: A justification for conservative operation. Ann. Surg., 158:37-46, 1963.

24. Patey, DH, and Dyson, WH. The prognosis of carcinoma of the breast in relation to the type of operation performed. Brit. J. Cancer, 2:7-13, 1948.

25. Nissen-Meyer, R. The role of prophylactic castration in therapy of human mammary cancer. Eur. J. Cancer, 3: 395-403, 1967.

26. Ravdin, RG, Lewison, EF, and Slack, NH, et al. Results of a clinical trial concerning the worth of prophylactic oophorectomy for breast carcinoma. Surg. Gynec. Obstet., 131:1055-1064, 1970.

27. Kim, K, Tidrick, RT, and Skeel, RT, et al. Fibrosarcoma of the chest wall following mastectomy and radiation therapy for mammary carcinoma. Breast, 6:1, pp. 26-30, Jan.-Mar. 1980.

28. Bittner, JJ. Some possible effects of nursing on the mammary gland tumor incidence in mice. Science, 84:162, 1936.

29. Romsdahl, MM, Sears, NE, and Eckles, NE. Closed-treatment evaluation of breast cancer. In Breast Cancer, Early and Late. Chicago: Year Book Medical Publishers, 1970, pp. 291-299.

Chapter 9

PREGNANCY AND CARDIOTHORACIC DISEASE

J. Terrance Davis, M.D.

INTRODUCTION

A consideration of the coexistence of pregnancy and cardiothoracic disease actually divides into two different points of
view, depending on which situation is complicating and which
is pre-existent. On one hand, a pregnant patient may develop
cardiothoracic disease requiring diagnostic and therapeutic
intervention during the pregnancy. In this situation, it is basically the cardiothoracic problem which is being managed and
the pregnancy adds a new dimension to the treatment. On the
other hand, a patient with established cardiothoracic disease
(for example, with a prosthetic cardiac valve in place) may become pregnant. Here the management of the pregnancy and delivery is the salient point, and the underlying alteration of cardiothoracic physiology adds interest to the management.

ACQUIRED CARDIAC DISEASE REQUIRING
TREATMENT DURING PREGNANCY

We will first consider the patient who in the course of pregnancy develops significant cardiac symptomatology. Pregnancy
is a substantial physiologic stress and may precipitate symptomatology in patients with cardiac disease which was previously
asymptomatic. On the other hand, cardiac disease may arise
de novo in the pregnant patient. Valvular heart disease is the
most common situation requiring operative intervention with
open heart surgery during pregnancy. Valvular heart disease
is usually rheumatic but may be on the basis of bacterial endocarditis and even acute aortic dissection. (1, 5)

No matter what the etiology, the problems posed by the necessity for open heart surgery and valve replacement in pregnancy are considerable. (5) The earliest reported use of extracorporeal circulation during pregnancy was in 1965. (2) Twenty such cases were reviewed in 1968. (3) The entire area was recently further reviewed and updated. (4) Several points have become clear as experience increased in this area. If at all possible the first and third trimesters should be avoided, and the best results are most likely going to be obtained in the second trimester. During the first trimester organogenesis is occurring, and the fetal mortality is probably in the range of 33%. During the third trimester difficulty with premature labor is a theoretical problem, although successful procedures have been reported as late as the thirty-second week of gestation. (6) Within the second trimester, cardiac surgery should be undertaken as early as possible. The physiologic stresses on the heart are maximum in the range of the thirtieth week and is the time when the patient is most likely to require definitive surgical help. Bacterial endocarditis requiring surgery cannot be timed with respect to the pregnancy and must be treated at such time as it is required because of cardiac decompensation.

Several technical points warrant emphasis. Monitoring of the fetal heart rate as well as the uterine contractions are mandatory. All reports include fetal bradycardia down to the range of 90 beats/minute as a baseline, probably related to moderate hypothermia. Bradycardia below this point is usually treated successfully by increasing the amount of cardiopulmonary bypass flow. Transient fetal tachycardia easily follows the restoration of maternal normal circulation. It is axiomatic that the shortest possible perfusion time, and highest possible perfusion flow rate will minimize the fetal risk.

Uterine contractions may occur during bypass, and some authors have recommended the use of intraoperative intravenous alcohol to suppress contractions(1) while others have recom-. mended no specific therapy. (4) Because of the small volume of cases presented to date and the large span of time over which they have been presented, meaningful maternal and fetal mortality figures are hard to gather. Mitral valvotomy or commissurotomy appear to carry a 2-3% maternal mortality and 9-12% fetal mortality. (7) Valve replacement would be expected to be somewhat higher, although not probably as high as the 5% maternal and 33% fetal mortality reported from the earlier collected series. (3)

It would seem wise to consider the use of the porcine valve in patients requiring valve replacement during pregnancy because of the likelihood of future pregnancy and the clear advantage of the biologic prosthesis with respect to anticoagulation, which will be discussed in a later section.

In summary, acquired valvular heart disease occasionally does require valve replacement with extracorporeal circulation even during pregnancy. Although there is risk in these procedures, both to the mother and fetus, the maternal risk does not appear to be undue with respect to the same procedure in non-pregnant patients. While there is substantial risk to the fetus, a normal live birth can certainly be expected in 75% of the cases or greater given proper attention to special monitoring techniques during the course of the procedure.

Coronary Artery Disease During Pregnancy

At the present time it is rare for coronary artery disease and pregnancy to coexist. While females in this age group are by and large protected from coronary artery disease by virtue of the hormonal environment, it is generally acknowledged that coronary artery disease does appear to be presenting in younger and younger age groups, even in females. In rare situations, where myocardial infarction occurs in the pregnant patient, if it occurs in the pregnant patient in the last trimester, the event is usually fatal. Survivors of the initial episode generally will tolerate labor and delivery. (46) It has been recommended, however, that the strain of labor and delivery should be avoided and elective caesarean section accomplished under these circumstances. (28)

It would seem predictable that at some time in the future a pregnant patient will present with symptomatic left main coronary artery disease or an equivalent situation mandating coronary artery bypass graft. To our knowledge there are no cases currently reported in this category, but the operative considerations should be essentially the same as those for valve replacement. In the situation of coronary artery bypass grafting, of course the postoperative anticoagulation would not be required and this would be one less area of concern.

Congenital Heart Disease Requiring Surgery During Pregnancy

Although congenital heart disease does not arise during pregnancy by definition, the symptomatology may be aggravated by the increased demand for cardiac output which peaks just before the thirtieth week and remains high for the remainder of the pregnancy, until just prior to parturition. In addition, the lowered systemic resistance may aggravate right-to-left shunting and cause an increase in cyanosis. Ordinarily, one may be carried medically through a pregnancy with an eye toward correction of one's underlying lesion at a later date. Details of this management are discussed later in the chapter. However, occasionally symptomatology increases to the point that open correction of the lesions must be undertaken.

The reported maternal mortality of 13% and fetal mortality of 40% are both quite high compared to the nonpregnant mortalities in these lesions. (8, 9) However, the numbers are small and recent data is lacking on this point and recent improvements in techniques may lead to better current results. General principles of anesthetic and surgical management as outlined in the previous section on cardiac surgery in patients with acquired cardiac disease apply to congenital disease as well. In addition to the risks outlined previously, the right-to-left shunting in many congenital diseases requires additional attention to the potential for a paradoxical embolus and for sudden desaturation because of changes in amount and direction of shunting at the cardiac level.

Arrhythmias Requiring Treatment During Pregnancy

Although many arrhythmias undoubtedly occur during the gestational period, most are benign. On occasion, however, severe arrhythmias may require defibrillation, and these have been reported with success. Ventricular fibrillation related to myocardial infarction(10) as well as atrial flutter(11) and refractory paroxysmal atrial tachycardia(12) have all been reported with successful cardioversion during pregnancy.

Medical management of these arrhythmias is clearly preferable to direct current countershock. The cardiac galactosides have not been shown to be teratogenic or in any other way harmful to the fetus. (13) Beta blockers on the other hand cross the placenta and therefore also can block the fetal adrenergic nervous system. The consequences include neonatal respiratory depression and hypoglycemia as well as increased uterine contraction, which may add to the risk of miscarriage. (14) Quinidine as an oxytocic stimulant has been considered contraindicated in the past during pregnancy. However, this is a controversial point and many now consider that in therapeutic doses, quinidine may be administered safely without fear of terminating the pregnancy. (15)

Pulmonary Disease Requiring Surgery During Pregnancy

While most thoracic lesions during pregnancy are predomi-
nantly medical and do not require operative intervention, pregnancy is not considered a major contraindication to whatever

intrathoracic work is required on the lungs. (16) A series of 29 pregnant women undergoing major thoracic procedures ranging from wedge resections through pneumonectomies has been reviewed. (17) No maternal deaths were noted in this series, and only one miscarriage followed a pneumonectomy. Procedures were performed for the usual spectrum of pulmonary disease. Carcinoma of the lung, when it becomes apparent during pregnancy, appears to be a rapidly progressive disease, and surgical intervention may not be warranted because of systemic spread at the time of original diagnosis. (18) The effect of successfully resected lung disease on the management and course of subsequent pregnancies is discussed in a later section.

Pulmonary trauma should be handled in accordance with the usual principles of management with particular attention to the avoidance of hypoxia. (16)

Pulmonary Embolism During Pregnancy

It is well known that pregnancy is a hypercoagulable state similar to other situations such as with patients on estrogen therapy, postoperative or post-traumatic patients, as well as patients with malignacies. (20) Therefore it is not surprising that thrombosis and thromboembolism occur with sufficient frequency to warrant concern, and some suggest the incidence is increasing. (19) The diagnosis of thromboembolism is made in the usual fashion including the standard procedures of electrocardiography and x-rays with due regard to the fetal well-being. Doppler ultrasound is helpful and can be done without fetal risk. Radioactive scanning techniques are not suitable for use in pregnancy since radioactive iodine crosses the placenta and is concentrated in the fetal thyroid gland. (20)

Assuming adequate documentation of thromboembolism, the question of therapy comes up. The use of anticoagulants in pregnant patients is discussed fully in a later section dealing with patients with prosthetic valves in place who are undergoing pregnancy. Suffice it to say here that oral warfarin derivatives are generally not indicated in these situations because of their teratogenicity and the high incidence of fetal hemorrhage. Heparin with its high molecular weight does not cross the placenta and is a useful drug in this situation for prevention of further thromboembolism. (21) It actually has been recommended as a prophylactic agent in patients with a strong history of previous embolization who have become pregnant. Recurrent embolus could be treated with the insertion of a Mobin-Uddin umbrella catheter in patients with recurrent embolism under adequate anticoagulation. However, to our knowledge this has not been reported in pregnancy, and the x-ray verification of position, which would be required would be of concern in the early stages of pregnancy.

Vena caval ligation could be accomplished without any exposure to x-ray with the usual risks of general anesthesia, which should be relatively small in this situation. Risk versus benefits of both approaches needs to be weighed in the individual patient.

Esophageal and Diaphragmatic Problems Requiring Surgery During Pregnancy

Hiatal Hernia

Hiatal hernia is a troublesome condition frequently aggravated by pregnancy. (16) This generally responds to the usual medical regimen of antacids, small frequent meals, and elevation of the head of the bed. Operative management ordinarily is not indicated.

However, diaphragmatic hernia in other areas, such as the Bochdalek hernia, appears to carry a high mortality when associated with strangulation during pregnancy. (22) Because of these alarming results, even though they are reported from earlier series, it is currently recommended that diaphragmatic hernias be repaired if discovered during pregnancy to prevent strangulation. (16)

Miscellaneous Thoracic Disorders Requiring Surgery During Pregnancy

A wide variety of disease entities may occur during pregnancy and be exacerbated by the pregnant state. Surgery may be required in certain instances.

An extensive procedure was reported during pregnancy in the first trimester to remove a thoracic vertebrae with partial pulmonary resection of a lung for radio-resistant giant cell tumor of the spine. In this situation the pregnancy was electively terminated after the surgery to prevent paraplegia. (23) Guillain-Barre syndrome has been reported in pregnancy, and tracheostomies have been required in certain cases. (24) Major reconstruction of the larynx has been reported in a patient of six months duration of pregnancy who sustained laryngeal trauma and disruption of the larynx. The pregnancy was carried to term successfully following reconstructive surgery on the larynx.

Myasthenia gravis is frequent in young females, and the pregnancy can coexist. Associated weakness and respiratory symptoms can complicate the pregnancy, but thymectomy has not to date been reported during pregnancy. It is noted that the infants of myasthenic mothers will have myasthenic symptoms lasting about six weeks which need to be anticipated in the neonatal unit. (26) It has been recommended, however, that recently married women with prospective hopes of children be considered for thymectomy in the hope that this will eliminate or decrease symptomatology in the mother and decrease difficulties with the neonate and myasthenic symptoms. (27)

MANAGEMENT AND PROGNOSIS OF PREGNANCY IN PATIENTS WITH INTRATHORACIC DISEASE

Pregnancy in the Patient with Acquired Heart Disease

Cardiac disease is present in approximately 0.5-2% of all pregnant females, and its management presents special challenges. (28) It is well known that pregnancy causes an increase in cardiac output which steadily rises during the early period of pregnancy, peaking at the thirtieth week and remaining high at that level until just before parturition. This is secondary to the effects of estrogen and progesterone on maternal cardiovascular function as well as the effects of the placental circulation. In both cases the peripheral resistance is decreased and a physiologic arteriovenous fistula is created by the circuit in parallel with the maternal circuit. (29) Digitalis and diuretics may be necessary to prevent heart failure in marginal situations. It is in these marginal situations where the maintenance of sinus rhythm becomes even more important because of its enhanced filling of the left ventricle and booster function.

In the case of unreplaced valvular heart disease, prophylaxis against bacterial endocarditis is recommended throughout pregnancy. Prophylaxis against rheumatic fever also should be kept in mind in those situations because recurrence can cause further damage.

Patients with prosthetic heart valves previously implanted present special problems. In most mechanical prostheses, anticoagulation is required to prevent systemic embolization. However, the hazards of anticoagulation are great and result in a significant fetal morbidity and mortality as well as maternal morbidity. Because of the relatively low molecular weight of warfarin derivatives, the placenta does not present a barrier and the fetus is presented with the drug. Within the first trimester it has long been recognized that coumarin is a teratogenic agent. (30, 31) In addition, coumarin is associated with a high risk of fetal intracerebral hemorrhage and hemorrhage in the mother. (32) Therefore, during the first and third trimester coumarin derivatives are to be avoided, and most recommend subcutaneous heparin for prevention of valve thrombosis. Heparin, because of its higher molecular weight, does not cross the placenta and is therefore safe for the fetus. In addition, it is more rapidly reversible and consequently more appropriate for management of the gravid situation.

Infective endocarditis on prosthetic cardiac valves is a risk of some magnitude. Prophylaxis for bacterial endocarditis should be undertaken in these patients during delivery and during any other invasive procedures or those which would predictably cause septicemia. Systemic embolization should immediately cause suspicion as to the current status of the valve.

Anesthetic considerations of management of delivery in patients with cardiac valves replaced are many. These have been cited in a number of articles(28,34) and need not be reviewed here. Suffice it to say that a thromboembolism must be avoided, additional cardiac output requirements must be met, and bacterial seeding of the prosthetic valve must be prevented or properly treated. The handling of labor is controversial. Some say that bearing down as part of labor is an additional demand on cardiac output which can be circumvented by using general anesthesia. Others feel that vaginal delivery with local anesthesia is preferable to caesarean section in cases of patients with prosthetic valves in place. (33)

Even with optimal medical, surgical, and anesthetic management (which has reduced maternal mortality to essentially that of normal pregnancy), fetal wastage remains high. Fetal mortality and morbidity range from 20 to 40% even with the best of techniques. (35-38) Nonetheless, in individual cases successful pregnancies bearing normal children have come about after prosthetic aortic valve replacement with complete heart block, (39) mitral valve replacement for infective endocarditis, (40) double valve replacement, (34) and triple valve replacement. (41) Successful pregnancy has even been reported following a near fatal thrombosis on a Bjork-Shiley valve. (42)

It is apparent that most of the difficulties with regard to pregnancy in patients with prosthetic valves relate to the use of warfarin derivatives. This has led many to favor the use of porcine xenograft valves in female patients of childbearing age because of the lack of necessity for anticoagulation in these valves. (44, 45)

Discussion of options with female patients with implanted heart valves needs to include both the fact that sterilization would of course prevent the problems of pregnancy but should also include the fact that normal healthy children are possible even with the most complex maternal cardiac situation.

Pregnancy in Patients with Congenital Heart Disease

Progress in both the medical and surgical management of congenital heart disease is creating a new population of patients who are just now moving in large numbers into the childbearing age and will be requiring information and management.

In general it may be stated that in congenital heart disease which has been corrected and where normal hemodynamics have been restored and there is no intracardiac shunting, the risk to mother and fetus are essentially minimal. It is only necessary to consider the somewhat higher incidence of heart disease among progeny of patients with congenital heart disease as opposed to the general population. The situation is substantially different, however, in uncorrected congenital heart disease where maternal and fetal risks rise dramatically.

Even so, patients with lesions characterized by predominantly left-to-right shunting do relatively well. Following the usual guidelines for management of such patients, (13) including elastic support to the legs, prophylactic antibiotic therapy, moderate diuresis, supplemental iron, and close follow-up, these patients will do relatively well. This is because with the initial problem being left-to-right shunting the cardiac output has a reasonable reserve in most cases. However, in situations in congenital lesions characterized by intracardiac right-to-left shunting, the situation is quite different. Here the alterations in maternal hemodynamics, particularly the decrease to peripheral resistance offered by the placenta, can cause an increase in right-to-left shunting and cyanosis.

The degree of right-to-left shunting in cyanotic heart disease is reflected by the maternal hematocrit and, in fact, patients with a maternal hematocrit of 65% or greater have a 75% chance of the pregnancy not going to term and ending in abortion. (28) In some conditions, such as Eisenmenger's syndrome and primary pulmonary hypertension with substantial cyanosis, maternal mortalities may run as high as 25-50%. (47) Anesthetic considerations in these situations are quite specific and have been well reviewed elsewhere. (28)

Certain other congenital situations are associated with relatively high maternal mortality as well as fetal wastage. These have been reviewed elsewhere, (13) but a few comments are worthwhile repeating here.

Coarctation of the aorta is unusual to remain unoperated into the childbearing years since the advent of modern cardiothoracic surgery. However, past experience has demonstrated that uncomplicated coarctation is compatible with a relatively uncomplicated pregnancy, labor, and delivery. However, complicated coarctation where maternal hypertension is a factor has a relatively high maternal mortality which may result from aortic rupture, acute congestive heart failure, cerebral vascular accidents, or bacterial endocarditis. Principles of the management of the pregnancy and treatment of parturition include avoidance of any additional increase in cardiac output other than what is absolutely necessary and specific prophylaxis for bacterial endocarditis, particularly if a vaginal delivery is employed.

Marfan's syndrome also is accompanied by a relatively high maternal mortality, including rupture of the aorta during pregnancy. Propranolol has been recommended to minimize aortic trauma during the third trimester and parturition.

Tetralogy of Fallot, as well as other lesions with high impedance to pulmonary blood flow, are susceptible to increased right-to-left shunting at various points during pregnancy and parturition. Diminution of venous return from factors such as supine hypotension in anesthesia as well as blood loss can exacerbate the situation. Parturition is the most dangerous time for these patients, and the cardiac output must be jealously maintained.

Cardiomyopathies, on the other hand, appear to be relatively well tolerated during pregnancy and parturition, and no major difficulties were reported in a series of 18 patients with obstructive cardiomyopathy carried through 22 pregnancies. (48) Propranolol was used to treat these patients and special care to prevent excessive or rapid blood loss resulting in a reduction in left heart volume and a subsequent increase in obstruction.

At the present time, with advances in the treatment of congenital heart disease, relatively special problems during pregnancy and parturition are being created. For instance, treatment of the tricuspid atresia and univentricular heart by atrial pulmonary connections leaves pulmonary blood flow to be propelled by vis a terga from the left ventricle without the aid of right ventricular contraction. How these patients will fare when faced with the stress of pregnancy is unknown at the present time. This and many other questions remain to be answered and constitute a fruitful area for future investigation.

Pregnancy in Patients Following Pulmonary Resection

It has been shown that following pulmonary resection ranging from segmental resection to pneumonectomy the potential for successful pregnancy is very much dependent on the prepregnancy condition of the patient with respect to respiratory reserve. In patients where there is no physical limitation or where dyspnea was created by only moderate or severe exercise, pregnancy and delivery may be expected to be essentially normal. (49) On the other hand, if dyspnea is caused by only mild exercise or is present at rest, maternal and fetal mortality rise. In addition to the problem of decreased available oxygen-carrying content for the fetus and subsequent fetal wastage, there is a significant incidence of reactivation or progression of native maternal disease under these circumstances. Termination of pregnancy has been recommended under these circumstances. It should be noted that the vast majority of patients fell into the asymptomatic or minimal symptomatic group, however. More recent data suggest that even after pneumonectomy, if this is performed for nonprogressive disease, that pregnancy is associated with an essentially normal outlook. (50)

REFERENCES

1. Werch, A, Lamber, HM, Cooley, D, and Reed, CC. Fetal monitoring and maternal open heart surgery. (Letters) Southern Med. J., 70:1024, 1977.

2. Ueland, K. Cardiac surgery and pregnancy. Am. J. Obstet. Gynecol., 92:148, 1965.

3. Zitnik, R, Brandenburg, R, Sheldon, R, et al. Pregnancy and open heart surgery. Circulation, 39:257, 1969.

4. Eilen, B, Kaiser, IH, Becker, RM, and Cohen, MN. Aortic valve replacement in the third trimester of pregnancy: Case report and review of the literature. Obstet. Gynecol., 57: 119, 1981.

5. Nazarian, M, McCullough, GH, and Fiedler, DL. Bacterial endocarditis in pregnancy: Successful surgical correction. J. Thorac. Cardiovas. Surg., 71:880, 1976.

6. Bahary, CM, Nimio, A, Gorodesky, IG, and Neri, A. Tococardiography in pregnancy during extracorporeal bypass for mitral valve replacement. Isr. J. Med. Sci., 16:395, 1980.

7. Kammerer, WS. Nonobstetric surgery during pregnancy. Med. Clin. N. Am., 63:1157, 1979.

8. Griffen, WO, Dilts, PV, and Roddick, JW. Current Problems in Surgery. Non-Obstetric Surgery During Pregnancy. Chicago, Year Book Medical Publishers, pp. 1-56, 1969.

9. Whittemore, R, and Hobbins, JC. Pregnancy in women who have congenital heart defects. Primary Cardiol., 3:26, 1977.

10. Curry, JJ, and Quintana, FJ. Myocardial infarction with ventricular fibrillation during pregnancy treated by direct current defibrillation with fetal survival. Chest, 58:82, 1970.

11. Sussman, H. Atrial flutter with 1:1 conduction successfully treated with DC shock. Dis. Chest, 49:99, 1966.

12. Schroeder, JS, and Harrison, DC. Repeated cardioversion during pregnancy. Treatment of refractory paroxysmal atrial tachycardia during 3 successive pregnancies. Am. J. Cardiol., 27:445, 1971.

13. Ueland, K. Cardiovascular diseases complicating pregnancy. Clin. Obstet. Gynecol., 21:429, 1978.

14. Heikila, J, Jounela, A, Katila, M, Ludmanmak, IK, and Frick, MH. Beta-blockade — selection and use. Ann. Clin. Res., 11:267 (Review), 1979.

15. Aviado, DM, and Salem, H. Drug action, reaction and interaction. I. Quinidine for cardiac arrhythymias. J. Clin. Pharmacol., 15:477, 1975.

16. Griffen, Jr., WO, Dilts, Jr., PV, and Roddick, Jr., JW. Non-obstetric surgery during pregnancy. Current Probl. Surg., pp. 1-56 (Review), 1969.

17. Tarnoff, J, Less, WM, and Fox, RT. Major thoracic surgery during pregnancy. Am. Rev. Resp. Dis., 96:1169, 1967.

18. Kennedy, A. Lung cancer in young adults. Br. J. Dis. Chest, 66:147, 1972.

19. Henderson, SR, et al. Antepartum pulmonary embolism. Am. J. Obstet. Gynecol., 112:476, 1972.

20. Barnett, HJ. Platelet and coagulation function in relation to thromboembolic stroke. Adv. Neurol., 16:45 (Review), 1977.

21. DeSwiet, M. Management of thromboembolism in pregnancy. Drugs, 18:478 (Review), 1979.

22. Penman, WR. Hiatus hernia. A cause of persistent gastrointestinal disturbances in pregnancy. West J. Surg., 59:622, 1951.

23. Larsson, SE. Removal of the third thoracic vertebra and partial lung resection for radioresistant giant-cell tumor of the spine. J. Bone Joint Surg. (Br.), 61:489, 1979.

24. Elstein, M, Legg, NJ, Murphy, M, Park, DM, and Sutcliffe, MM. Guillian-Barre syndrome in pregnancy. Respiratory paralysis complicated by a fatal tracheo-innominate artery fistula. Anaesthesia, 26:216, 1971.

25. Desanto, LW, Brown, Jr., AK, Acute laryngeal trauma. Its early management. Minn. Med., 55:328, 1972.

26. Ryan, M, Egbert, B, and Ziebler, DK. Myasthenia gravis and immunity. A review of basic mechanisms. J. Kans. Med. Soc., 74:72, 1973.

27. Edwards, FR, and Wilson, A. Thymectomy for myasthenia gravis. Thorax, 27:513, 1972.

28. Ostheimer, GW, and Alper, MH. Intrapartum anesthetic management of the pregnant patient with heart disease. Clin. Obstet. Gynecol., 18:81, 1975.

29. McCans, JL, and Wenger, NK. Problems in management of the pregnant patient with rheumatic heart disease and valve prosthesis. Southern Med. J., 69:1007, 1976.

30. Oakley, C, and Doherty, P. Pregnancy in patients after valve replacement. Br. Heart J., 38:1140, 1976.

31. Murphy, ES, and Kloster, FE. Late results of valve replacement surgery. II. Complications of prosthetic heart valves. Mod. Concepts Cardiovasc. Dis., 48:59, 1959.

32. Alby, AJ, Stevens, JE, and Beck, W. The clinical assessment and management of patients with prosthetic cardiac valves: A review of current practice at the cardiac clinic, Groote Schuur Hospital. S. HFR Med. J., 57:307, 1980.

33. Saka, DM, and Marx, GF. Management of a parturient with cardiac valve prosthesis. Anesth. Analg. (Cleve.), 55:214, 1976.

34. Gothard, JW. Heart disease in pregnancy. The anesethetic management of a patient with prosthetic heart valves. Anaesthesia, 33:523, 1978.

35. Tejani, N. Anticoagulant therapy with cardiac valve prosthesis during pregnancy. Obstet. Gynecol., 42:785, 1973.

36. Buxbaum, A, Aygen, MM, Shahin, W, Levy, MJ, and Ekerling, B. Pregnancy in patients with prosthetic heart valves. Chest, 59:639, 1971.

37. Vidne, B, Erdman, S, and Levy, MJ. Thromboembolism following heart valve replacement by prosthesis: Survey among 365 consecutive patients. Chest, 63:713, 1973.

38. Harrison, EC, and Roschke, EJ. Pregnancy in patients with cardiac valve protheses. Clin. Obstet. Gynecol., 18:107, 1975.

39. Bemiller, CR, Forker, AD, and Morgan, JR. Complete heart block, prosthetic aortic valves and successful pregnancy. JAMA, 214:915, 1970.

40. Yacoub, M, Pennacchio, L, Ross, D, and McDonald, L. Replacement of mitral valve in active infective endocarditis. Br. Heart J., 34:758, 1972.

41. Nagorney, DM, and Field, CS. Successful pregnancy 10 years after triple cardiac valve replacement. Obstet. Gynecol., 57:386, 1981.

42. McLeod, AA, Jennings, KP, and Townsend, ER. Near fatal puerperal thrombosis of Bjork-Shiley mitral valve prosthesis. Br. Heart J., 40:934, 1978.

43. Kirklin, JW. The replacement of cardiac valves (Editorial). N. Engl. J. Med., 304:291, 1981.

44. Editorial: Pregnancy after valve replacement. Lancet, 1:462, 1976.

45. Beadle, Jr., EM, Leupker, RV, and William, PP. Pregnancy in a patient with porcine valve xenografts. Am. Heart J., 98:510, 1979.

46. Husaini, MH. Myocardial infarction during pregnancy: Report of two cases with a review of the literature. Postgrad. Med. J., 47:660, 1971.

47. Rowland, TW. The pediatrician and congenital heart disease — 1979. Pediatrics, 64:180 (Review), 1979.

48. Turner, GM, Oakley, CM, and Dixon, HG. Management of pregnancy complicated by hypertrophic obstructive cardiomyopathy. Br. Med. J., 4:281-284, 1968.

49. Tandon, RK, Patney, NC, Goyal, SP, and Tandon, K. Pulmonary resection in child bearing age and its effect on pregnancy. Indian J. Chest Dis., 16:381, 1974.

50. Laros, KD. The postpneumonectomy mother. Pregnancy, delivery and motherhood. 80 patients followed through more than 20 years after surgery. Respiration, 39:185, 1980.

Chapter 10

THE MANAGEMENT OF HERNIAS DURING PREGNANCY

Hollis W. Merrick, M.D.

Hernias that require surgical intervention during pregnancy
are rare. The magnitude of this problem is not apparent in a
review of the literature, as these hernias either do not present
a problem or are not often reported. In two series from the
1940s which report incidences, (1, 2) in over 100, 000 pregnancies
only four patients with hernias required surgery during pregnancy because of incarceration. Nonetheless, a wide variety of
hernias have been reported to occur during pregnancy and can
pose serious danger to the mother and fetus. The presence of
a hernia requires **close** observation of the patient, as an unrec-
ognized complication can be fatal.

The symptoms of early obstruction or strangulation can be
similar to commonly occurring functional or gastrointestinal
disturbances of pregnancy. Pregnancy does not change the symptoms of a hernia, but the increased intra-abdominal pressure
associated with the third trimester of pregnancy may **aggravate**
these symptoms. A diagnosis of strangulating bowel obstruction
requires prompt operation and takes precedence over other considerations of the pregnancy. The maternal mortality rate for a
strangulated hernia during pregnancy varies from 25 to 88%. (3)
The question of elective repair of hernias during pregnancy depends upon the danger that the type of hernia poses but should
probably be limited to those hernias with evidence of incarceration.

Classification
External
    Femoral
    Inguinal
    Umbilical
    Ventral (incisional)
    Diastasis recti

Internal
   Diaphragmatic
     Congenital (Bochdalek)
     Hiatal
     Post-traumatic
   Pelvic
     Broad ligament
     Obturator
     Sciatic
     Lumbar
     Gynecologic

EXTERNAL HERNIAS

Abdominal wall hernias occur far less frequently in women than in men. Despite femoral hernias being more common in females, they are only half as common as indirect inguinal hernias in males. The female abdominal wall is very resistant to hernia formation despite obesity, pregnancy, and multiple surgeries. (4)

The differences in incidence of external hernias between the sexes is accounted for by variations in embryology and anatomy. The descent of the testis with the scrotum results in a definite weakness in the male groin. In the female the distal portion of the round ligament extends to the labia majoris. Invagination of peritoneum to the round ligament is known as the canal of Nuck. This structure is usually obliterated by the eighth fetal month, but should it persist an indirect inguinal hernia could result. The transversalis fascia and transversus abdominus are well-developed layers in the female. Direct hernias through Hesselbach's triangle are uncommon. McVay(5) has indicated that the attachment of the transversus abdominus to Cooper's ligament is important in preventing direct and femoral hernias. The angle between Cooper's ligament and inguinal ligament is less in females due to structural differences in the female pelvis. However, the interval between the medial aspect of the femoral ring and the femoral vein is larger in females and may help account for the increased occurrence of the femoral hernias.

Pregnancy changes the anatomical presentation of hernias and their management. With the enlargement of the uterus, there is increased intra-abdominal pressure resulting in increased pressure on the abdominal contents. There is, as well, a stretching of the abdominal wall which enlarges the hernia defect. Thus, hernias which were small and nonsymptomatic before pregnancy may become evident during pregnancy. The greater the degree of enlargement of the uterus and fetus, as associated with twins, the greater the incidence of complications.

Femoral and Inguinal Hernias

These hernias are only one-tenth as common in females as in males. (4) It was previously believed that femoral hernias were more common than inguinal hernias in females, but recent reports indicate that indirect inguinal hernias are twice as common as femoral hernias. Direct inguinal hernias are rare.

The groin hernias are usually symptomatic only during the first trimester. As the uterus enlarges along the anterior abdominal wall the bowel is displaced and the uterus occludes the hernia. If the bowel is adherent to the defect, strangulation may result as the uterus enlarges. The uterus can become incarcerated in a very large groin defect.

The diagnosis of a groin hernia may be easily overlooked, especially in an obese patient. A lump in the groin is not necessarily a hernia but can be a fibroma or myoma of the round ligament, dilated groin veins, or a hydrocele of the canal of Nuck. (6) An occurrence of a fibromatous nodule in a pregnant uterus simulating incarcerated inguinal hernia was reported. (7) Rupture of a varicose vein of the round ligament in pregnancy simulating a strangulated hernia also has been reported. (8) Indirect inguinal hernias in pregnant or postpartum females have been described without a palpable sac, presenting with unilateral groin pain. (9) Three case reports of ectopic pregnancies presenting in a groin hernia have been reported.(10-12) An unusual surgical emergency(13) has been reported to have occurred in the thirty-seventh week of pregnancy when a left inguinal hernia was found to contain one horn of the uterus, the round ligament, a fallopian tube, and an ovary. An incarcerated right ovary and fallopian tube in a groin hernia has also been reported. (14)

Hernias diagnosed in a young female should be repaired before pregnancy. These hernias usually should not be repaired during pregnancy, but should a complication occur, prompt surgical intervention is indicated. If no problems have arisen during pregnancy, the hernias should be repaired promptly postpartum as they may well increase in size and symptoms. Bowel that is adherent to a hernial sac is liable to injury at any time but most significantly during the second stage of labor when the intra-abdominal pressure is maximally increased. During delivery, the decreased size of the uterus may again allow entry of bowel into a defect, and the patient must be watched closely for incarceration. If a groin hernia does not reduce in the second trimester or if a history of prior incarceration is present, elective repair of the hernia is probably the safest course.

Umbilical Hernias

Umbilical hernias are usually small and asymptomatic. They do not usually incarcerate after the sixth month of pregnancy because the uterus becomes a barrier to the bowel. However, such hernias commonly contain adherent omentum which may cause symptoms. It is advisable to repair a nonreducible hernia before the enlarging uterus causes possible strangulation. After the delivery, the hernial defect is likely to have become larger and repair, especially if another pregnancy is likely, is indicated. Umbilical incarceration of the uterus at term requiring emergency caesarean section has been reported. (15-19) Ulceration of the skin with actual rupture of the hernia during labor has been reported by de Glanville(20) and Young. (21) Interestingly, both patients suffered rupture during the seventh month of pregnancy. Castleden(22) reported a ruptured umbilical hernia containing a Meckel's diverticulum.

Ventral Hernias

Ventral hernias may first become evident during the course of pregnancy. The change in size of the uterus with accompanying increase in intra-abdominal pressure can enlarge previous defects or cause new ones in poorly healed incisions. They are usually seen in vertical lower abdominal incisions secondary to obstetrical and gynecological procedures. These hernias usually have a broad neck and uncommonly cause obstruction and strangulation. Abdominal support is indicated during delivery, with shortened second stage by use of forceps. A postpartum repair is indicated. Fullman(23) reported the occurrence of twin pregnancy in an obese patient with a large incisional hernia which required an emergency caesarean section. Two additional cases have been reported of uterine incarceration in larger ventral defects. (24, 25)

Diastasis Recti

Diastasis recti is not strictly speaking a hernia. However, the rectus muscles may become separated to such a degree that it causes some discomfort in the last trimester and may severely compromise the ability of the patient to bear down during labor. During delivery the use of a binder and fundal pressure along with forceps delivery usually compensates for the defect. Rarely the diastasis may need to be repaired after the patient has finished her childbearing.

DIAPHRAGMATIC HERNIAS

Hiatal Hernias

Hiatal hernia is a frequent occurrence during pregnancy. Rigler and Eneboe(26) performed upper gastrointestinal tract radiographs in the last trimester on 195 patients. They found an incidence of hiatal hernia of 12.5%, with a higher incidence in multiparous mothers. Some of these patients were evaluated postpartum, and the hernias had disappeared. This was thought to be due to the role of increased intra-abdominal pressure during pregnancy. Although the hiatal hernia is the most common type found during pregnancy, the incidence of strangulation is low. It produces axial protrusion of the stomach into the chest, which rarely causes gangrene to occur. Because of their position, hiatal hernias almost never produce incarceration of the small or large bowel. (27)

Congenital Diaphragmatic Hernias

Bochdalek described a developmental defect in the diaphragm in which there was a persistence of the pleural-peritoneal canal. The defects are posterio-lateral, more common on the left, and typically do not have a hernia sac. The defects usually cause serious problems in the unborn but may not be manifested until adulthood. This is especially true in a period of increased intra-abdominal pressure, as in pregnancy. Other congenital defects, such as the retrosternal defect of Morgagni, have not been reported in the literature to cause problems in pregnancy.

Post-Traumatic Diaphragmatic Hernias

This type of hernia is caused by stab wounds or gunshot wounds to the diaphragm or by indirect trauma due to falls, compression injuries, or motor vehicle accidents. (28, 29) These hernias have shown a progressive increase in occurrence since World War I due to the increased trauma in our society. Wounds of the diaphragm are prone not to heal because negative pressure in the chest causes migration of intra-abdominal organs. A portion of omentum or an organ may plug the defect and separate the muscle fibers, preventing their union. The defect thus created remains a constant threat to the patient, particularly when pregnancy intervenes with a subsequent increase in intra-abdominal pressure.

Management of Diaphragmatic Hernias During Pregnancy

Congenital and traumatic diaphragmatic hernias are much less common than hiatal hernia during pregnancy, but the incidence of strangulation is extremely high. Penman(30) reviewed 13 cases, of which 11 were diaphragmatic and 2 were hiatal. Of the 11 patients with diaphragmatic hernias, 8 died; only 4 of these patients underwent surgical correction, and 3 survived. Both patients with hiatal hernias recovered without surgical correction.

Post-traumatic hernias have a high incidence of strangulation. Many authors(31-44) have found that 90% of the diaphragmatic hernias complicated by obstruction and strangulation were of the post-traumatic type. Congenital hernias are less common, but the incidence of strangulation is still high, as reported by numerous authors. (45-52) The intra-abdominal contents may reside in the lower section on the left chest. With increase in intra-abdominal pressure during pregnancy, there is a possibility of incarceration. Diaphragmatic hernias may be asymptomatic early in the pregnancy, but the onset of complaints in the second and third trimester of pregnancy should signal the possible presence of these hernias. The symptoms may consist of vague complaints of nausea and vomiting and the onset of left upper quadrant pain.

The physical findings can be mistaken for a pneumothorax because of the respiratory distress, absence of breath sounds, and tympany of the chest. A chest tube may be inadvertently introduced into the stomach or intestine as reported by Savage. (51) Chest x-rays usually demonstrate the presence of abdominal contents, and an air bubble behind the heart or an air-fluid level in the left chest is diagnostic. If the hernia is strangulated, there may be a pleural effusion or empyema(50) on the chest x-ray. Bowel obstruction may be manifested by crampy abdominal pain with nausea and vomiting. Respiratory distress and dullness to percussion of the chest also may be present. The presence of steady pain with the respiratory distress accompanied by left pleural effusion are indications of strangulation. These clinical findings during the third stage of labor or immediately postpartum should alert the physician to the possibility of this type of hernia. A patient with a known diaphragmatic hernia should not become pregnant unless the hernia is repaired.

If the presence of a diaphragmatic hernia is detected during pregnancy, the patient warrants close observation. The history of a prior normal delivery does not mean the patient will have an uncomplicated delivery.(37) The post-traumatic and congenital hernias are particularly prone to strangulation with a high mortality. Patients with known diaphragmatic hernia should not be allowed to go into labor. Because of the difficulty in making the diagnosis when the defect is small, barium enema or upper gastrointestinal radiography may be indicated in those patients with history of prior trauma. A caesarean section is indicated if evidence of obstruction occurs: immediate repair of the hernia also is indicated.

A patient with a hiatal hernia, however, may be followed through the period of labor and delivery with good nasogastric decompression and observation. If signs of impending obstruction develop, then immediate surgery is indicated. The risk of a complication from a diaphragmatic hernia is much greater than the risk of a caesarean section. If the patient in labor develops left upper quadrant pain, respiratory distress, hemotemesis, nausea, or vomiting, a diaphragmatic hernia should be suspected. A chest x-ray is usually diagnostic, and prompt caesarean section is indicated.

INTERNAL HERNIAS

Intra-Abdominal Hernias

Incarceration can occur through any internal defect in large or small bowel mesentery. Two recent reports(53, 54) describe herniation through the foramen of Winslow during the last trimester of pregnancy.

Broad Ligament Hernias

The broad ligament is susceptible to hernia defects developing after laceration during pregnancy, uterine suspension, or congenital anomalies. The small bowel may herniate through the defect, and although obstruction and strangulation are uncommon, they can occur.(55)

Obturator of Sciatic Hernias

The intestine may herniate through either an obturator foramen or a sciatic foramen. Obstruction is uncommon, but pain may develop in the area of the distribution of the obturator or sciatic nerves. Reduction and closure of the defect is indicated.

Levator Hernias

A levator hernia is a defect between the pubococcygeus and the ileococcygeus muscle on either side, which permits a herniation posteriorly into the perineum in front of the transverse peroneal muscle. An anterior defect may include the bladder and intestine. (56) These hernias do not cause problems in pregnancy unless the intestine is fixed to the defect and becomes strangulated as the uterus enlarges.

Gynecological Hernias

During delivery enteroceles or rectoceles may impede delivery if these defects are large. Treatment is by simple replacement of the prolapsed structure after each contraction, permitting the fetus to pass the bladder or rectal pouch. Emptying the bladder and rectum is mandatory before delivery.

SUMMARY

Complications in pregnancy due to hernias have not been perceived as a significant problem. However, the variety of hernias which may cause problems is extensive. The danger lies in overlooking the presence of a hernia and failing to diagnose a problem quickly when it occurs. The diaphragmatic hernias are particularly treacherous due to their insidious and rapid onset, commonly in the midst of the process of delivery. Hernias occurring during pregnancy require awareness of the potential problems, astuteness in diagnosis, and promptness in surgical therapy.

REFERENCES

1. Smith, JA, and Bartlett, MK. Acute surgical emergencies of the abdomen in pregnancy. N. Engl. J. Med., 223:529, 1940, p. 161-168.

2. Child III, CG, and Douglas, RG. Surgical problems arising during pregnancy. Am. J. Obstet. Gynecol., 47:213, 1944.

3. Kesseler, HJ. Hernias in pregnancy. In Surgical Disease in Pregnancy, Barber, HRK, and Garber, LA (Eds.). Philadelphia, W. B. Saunders Co., 1974, pp. 161-168.

4. Ponka, JL. The hernia problem in the female. In Hernias of the Abdominal Wall, Ponka, JL (Ed.). Philadelphia, W. B. Saunders Co., 1980, pp. 82-90.

5. McVay, CG. Christopher's Textbook of Surgery, 7th Ed. Philadelphia, W. B. Saunders Co., 1960, pp. 524-569.

6. Hodgkinson, CP, and Kroll, J. Inguinal swelling during pregnancy. Am. J. Obstet. Gynecol., 73:966, 1957.

7. Lysak, ZA. Fibromatous nodule in the pregnant uterus simulating incarcerated inguinal hernia. Rus. Klin. Khir., 2:82, 1978.

8. Blanda, F. Rupture of varicose veins of the round ligament in pregnancy simulating a strangulated hernia. Minerva Gynecol., 69(2):48-50, 1969.

9. Fodor, PB, and Webb, WA. Indirect inguinal hernia in the female with no palpable sac. Southern Med. J. 64(1): 15-16, 1971.

10. Surgarman, GR. Tubal pregnancy in hernia sac: Case report. J. Newark Beth Israel Hosp., 12:160, 1961.

11. D'Souza, R, and Richard, HL. Ectopic pregnancy in a hernia sac: A case report. Can. J. Surg., 13(2):166-167, 1970.

12. Polak, L, Witek, R, Bader, O, and Kibler, J. Case of ectopic pregnancy disclosed during inguinal herniotomy. Pol. Wiad. Lek., 27(16):1521-1523, 1974.

13. Mechacek, J, and Silhan, J. Right side ovarian and tubal incarceration through strangulation in pregnancy. Cesk. Gynekol., 43(9):717, 1978.

14. Mahmad, A. Unusual surgical emergency in pregnancy. Br. Med. J., 3(725):772, 1970.

15. Mays, ET. Eventration through umbilical hernia during pregnancy. J. Kentucky M.A., 67(2):110-112, 1969.

16. Boys, CE. Strangulated hernia containing pregnant uterus at term. Am. J. Obstet. Gynecol., 50:450, 1945.

17. Castro, NE. A pregnant uterus protruding through an umbilical hernial sac. S. Afr. Med. J. , 49(43):1774, 1975.

18. Zanke, S, and Adam, G. Large paraumbilical hernia and pregnancy. Case report. Ger. Zentralbl. Gynaekol. , 100(12):825-828, 1978.

19. Intrauterine pregnancy prolapse in umbilical hernia. Rev. Fr. Gynecol. Obstet. , 62(9):503-505, 1967.

20. de Glanville, H. Ruptured umbilical hernia. Lancet, 269: 1321, 1955.

21. Young, BK. Ruptured umbilical hernia in pregnancy. Report of a case. Obstet. Gynecol. , 26(4):596-598, 1965.

22. Castleden, WM. Meckel's diverticulum in an umbilical hernia. Br. J. Surg. , 57(12):932-934, 1970.

23. Fullman, PM. An incisional hernia containing an incarcerated twin pregnant uterus. Am. J. Obstet. Gynecol. , 111(2):308-309, 1971.

24. Azkowski, H, Mierzejewski, W, and Rudzininski, J. Development of pregnancy in a uterus located in a vast post-operative hernia complicated by placenta previa. Pol. Ginekol. Pol. , 48(4):395-397, 1977.

25. Usmandy, IAA. Strangulated uterus in a ventral hernia in the region of the linea allea. Rus. Kirurgiia. (Mosk), No. 8, pp. 125-126, 1977.

26. Rigler, LG, and Eneboe, JR. Incidence of hiatus hernia in pregnant women and its significance. J. Thorac. Surg. , 4:262, 1935.

27. Sprafka, JL, Azad, M, and Baronofsky, ID. Fate of esophageal hiatus hernia — A clinical and experimental study. Surgery, 36:3. 1954.

28. Mengert, WF, and Murphy, DP. Intra-abdominal pressures created by voluntary muscular effort. III. Relation to body measurements with comment on etiology of genital prolapse. Surg. Gynecol. Obstet. , 58:150, 1934.

29. Bushsbaum, HJ. Trauma in Pregnancy. Philadelphia, W. B. Saunders Co., 1979, pp. 104-112.

30. Penman, WR. Hiatal hernia: A cause of persistent gastrointestinal disturbances in pregnancy. West. J. Surg., 59: 622, 1951.

31. Carter, BN, and Giuseffi, J. Strangulated diaphragmatic hernia. Ann. Surg., 128:210, 1948.

32. Vijayanagar, R, and Hofstra, PC. Obstruction and strangulation in diaphragmatic hernia due to direct trauma. N. Y. J. Med., 71:1228, 1971.

33. Ebert, PA, Gaertner, RA, and Zuidema, GD. Traumatic diaphragmatic hernia. Surg. Gynecol. Obstet. 125:59, 1967.

34. Harrington, SW. Traumatic diaphragmatic hernia in pregnancy. Surg. Clin. N. Am., 30:961, 1950.

35. Sullivan, RE. Strangulation and obstruction in a diaphragmatic hernia due to trauma. Report of two cases and review of English literature. J. Thorac. Surg., 52:725, 1966.

36. DeLee, ST, and Gilson, BI. Diaphragmatic hernia complicating the peurperium. Am. J. Obstet. Gynecol. 41: 904, 1941.

37. Diddle, AW, and Tidrick, RT. Diaphragmatic hernia associated with pregnancy. Am. J. Obstet. Gynecol., 41:317, 1941.

38. Kushlan, SD. Diaphragmatic hernia in pregnancy: Significance and danger. Conn. Med. J., 15:969, 1951.

39. Shevchuk, MG, Serediuk, NN, Tkachuk, LI, Ostafiichuk, MI, and Furda, MD. Complicated diaphragmatic hernias. Rus. Klin. Med. (Mosk), 54(2):137-138, 1976.

40. Zimmermann, HD, and Stracke, H. Sudden maternal death in late pregnancy: Congenital diaphragmatic defect causing prolapse of the intestine into the thoracic cavity (author's translation). Ger. Gerburtshilfe Frauenheilkd, 37(10): 882-886, 1977.

41. Barnett, DS, Van Dongen, LGR, and Bremner, CG. Traumatic diaphragmatic hernia presenting in pregnancy. S. Afr. Med. J., 55(3):945, 1979.

42. Dudley, AG, Teafor, H, and Gatewood, TS. Delayed traumatic rupture of the diaphragm in pregnancy. Obstet. Gynecol. 53(3):22S-27S, 1979.

43. Bernhardt, LC. Pregnancy complicated by traumatic rupture of the diaphragm, Am. J. Surg., 112:918-922, 1966.

44. Kessler, E, and Stein, A. Diaphragmatic hernia as a long-term complication of stab wounds of the chest. Am. J. Surg., 132:34-39, 1976.

45. Thompson, JW, and LeBlane, LJ. Congenital diaphragmatic hernia: Visceral strangulation complicating delivery. Am. J. Surg., 67:123, 1945.

46. Pearson, SC. Strangulated diaphragmatic hernia complicating pregnancy. JAMA, 144:22, 1950.

47. Bourgeois, GA, and Hood, WT. Strangulated diaphragmatic hernia complicating pregnancy. N. Engl. J. Med., 241:150, 1949.

48. Browning, DJ. Maternal death and diaphragmatic hernia. Med. J. Australia, 2(6):297, 1973.

49. Carter, R, and Brewer, LA. Strangulating diaphragmatic hernia. Ann. Thorac. Surg., 12(3):281-290, 1971.

50. Golstein, AI, Gazzaniga, AB, Ackerman, ES, Rajcher, WJ, Kent, DR, and Campbell, R. Strangulated diaphragmatic hernia in pregnancy presenting as an empyema. J. Repro. Med. 9(3):135-139, 1972.

51. Savage, PT. Obstructed volvulus of the stomach in a diaphragmatic hernia; a post-partum emergency. Proc. R. Soc. Med., 61(10):956-958, 1968.

52. Tsakadze, LO, Moiseev, NV, and Butina, NP: Strangulated congenital diaphragmatic hernia in a patient in the 36th week of pregnancy. Rus. Vestn. Khir., 112(3):122-124, 1974.

53. Gneo, S. A case of hernia of the hiatus of Winslow in the 7th month of pregnancy. Anatomoclinical and surgical considerations. Ita Minerva Ginecol., 31(12):911-915, 1979.

54. Still, RM, and Scott, R. Hernia through the foramen of Winslow in pregnancy. J. Obstet. Gynecol. Br. Commonw., 74(6):939-940, 1967.

55. Kyosola, K. Simultaneous occurrence of ovarian torsion and gangrenous strangulation through a congenital opening in the mesosalpinx, Ann. Clin. Gynecol., 66(6):290-291, 1977.

56. Sotnichenko, BA. Perineal hernias, their diagnosis and treatment. Klin. Khir., 9:75, 1968.

Chapter 11

DRUG THERAPY DURING PREGNANCY

Pitambar Somani, M.D., and Daniel Brown, Pharm.D.

INTRODUCTION

Drug therapy decisions involving the pregnant patient generally warrant a number of careful considerations. Although the physician generally intends to prescribe these drugs to elicit the intended pharmacologic effects solely in the mother, in most cases the fetus is inadvertently exposed to the drug as well.

Recent concern regarding exposing the fetus to various drugs taken by the mother has resulted from the growing awareness of the potential teratogenic effects of many drugs, sometimes even years after the drug exposure, such as the occurrence of vaginal cancers with diethylstilbestrol. Highly sensitive techniques such as the GC-Mass Spectrography have also been used effectively to document the presence of various drugs in the amniotic fluid and fetal blood, even in utero, and such data clearly suggest that most, if not all, drugs can pass from the mother to the fetus through the placental circulation. It is, therefore, very important to take all necessary precautions when prescribing drugs to pregnant women.

Drug therapy during pregnancy requires several important practical considerations, especially with regards to the selection of an appropriate agent, adjustment of drug dosage, teratogenicity of certain drugs, toxic drug effects on fetal growth and function, and passage of drugs into the breast milk. Any surgeon dealing with pregnant patients should be fully aware of the serious risks involved in prescribing drugs to such patients, and in this chapter we will review these aspects of drug therapy, especially the problem of drug-induced fetal malformation or the so-called teratogenicity.

Over 600 chemicals, drugs, or viruses have produced teratogenicity in experimental animals, though only about 25 have been documented to cause human malformations. (1) However, any agent, when administered in sufficient dose during a critical period of gestation, may be a potential teratogen.

The overall incidence of major congenital malformations is approximately 2-3% of all births; however, the incidence of minor malformations may be as high as 9%. (2) It is alarming to note that only 2-3% of congenital defects are known to be definitely caused by drugs or environmental chemicals, whereas 65-70% of such birth defects are of unknown etiology. (3) Furthermore, pregnant women take an average of four drugs during the course of pregnancy, excluding nutritional supplements, (3) and therefore, a potentially serious health hazard exists for the newborn.

When evaluating the potential effect of a drug on the fetus, one must consider the dose and pharmacokinetic parameters of the drug, the extent of placental drug transfer, the effect of drug metabolites, and the stage of fetal development at the time of exposure. If a drug is suspected to have teratogenic potential, the clinician must weigh the anticipated maternal therapeutic benefit against possible fetal toxicity. As a general rule, it is best to avoid the use of all medications and recreational substances in pregnant patients.

Placental Drug Transfer

Drugs cross the placenta primarily via passive diffusion, although some active and facilitative transport processes do exist for certain drugs which can result in fetal drug accumulation against a concentration gradient. Generally, drugs with a gram-molecular-weight (GMW) of less than 500 g cross the placenta easily; those with a GMW of 500-1000 g cross it to a lesser extent, and those with a GMW greater than 1000 g do not cross the placenta. (4) The GMW of most drugs is in the range of 250-500 g.

The following factors affect the rate at which a drug crosses the placenta. (4)

1. pH
2. pKa of the drug
3. oil/water partition coefficient of the drug
4. area of maternal-fetal exchange
5. thickness of the decidual membrane
6. molecular weight of the drug
7. rates of maternal and placental blood flows
8. free (nonprotein-bound) drug concentration in maternal blood

The placenta is an organ which also is capable of drug metabolism, specifically those reactions involving oxidation, reduction, conjugation, and hydroxylation. The teratogenicity potential of a drug's metabolite may differ significantly from that of the parent drug, and therefore, by metabolizing a given drug the placenta itself may alter the teratogenicity of a given agent.

Embryonic and Fetal Development

The nature and extent of teratogenicity resulting from a specific agent are heavily dependent upon the timing of drug exposure during pregnancy. The most critical period is the first trimester of pregnancy, during which organogenesis takes place. Differentiation of the embryo begins during the second week of gestation and continues for approximately eight weeks. (2) During this period of organogenesis drugs may produce severe structural abnormalities, whereas defects resulting from the second or third trimester drug exposure are more likely to reflect abnormalities in growth or functional development. (2, 5) During the latter two trimesters, development of the central nervous system is particularly susceptible to teratogens, and defects are frequently manifested by microcephaly or mental retardation. (5)

Exposure to drugs in utero may also result in delayed effects, such as carcinogenesis, which become apparent in later life. (5)

Lastly, one must be aware that at birth, the neonate's capacity to metabolize or excrete drugs is poorly developed and therefore the neonate may be subjected to prolonged drug effect even though it was administered to the mother shortly before term. (5, 6) This is specially the case for most drugs, such as propranolol, whose metabolism depends upon enzymatic processes in the liver.

FDA Pregnancy Labeling Regulations

Due to a general lack of available information regarding the teratogenic potential of many prescription drugs, the FDA has established regulations for pregnancy labeling. These regulations, which were implemented in 1980, identified five pregnancy categories. (7, 8)

A. Controlled studies in women fail to demonstrate a risk to the fetus in the first trimester, and the possibility of fetal harm appears remote.

B.   Animal studies do not indicate a risk to the fetus and there are no controlled human studies; or animal studies do show an adverse effect on the fetus but well-controlled studies in pregnant women have failed to demonstrate a risk to the fetus.

C.   Studies have shown the drug to have animal teratogenic or embryonic effects, but there are no controlled studies in women, or no studies are available in either animals or women.

D.   Positive evidence of human fetal risk exists, but benefits in certain situations (i.e., life threatening situations or serious diseases for which safer drugs cannot be used or are ineffective) may make use of the drug acceptable during pregnancy despite its risks.

E.   Studies in animals or humans have demonstrated fetal abnormalities or there is evidence of fetal risk based on human experience, or both, and the risk clearly outweighs any possible benefit.

When evaluating a drug according to the above categories, one must consider that the data from animal studies alone may be misleading. Indeed, some teratogenic manifestations are species-specific. (9) One such example is the case of thalidomide, which was released in Europe in the late 1950s as a safe tranquilizer/hypnotic. Although initial animal studies failed to demonstrate congenital malformations, an estimated 10,000 children were eventually born with thalidomide-induced phacomelia. (9) Although it is impossible to review and discuss the teratogenic effects of all drugs in this chapter, we would summarize available data for several broad categories of drugs commonly used by surgeons.

ANALGESICS

Narcotics

Narcotic analgesics, such as meperidine or alphaprodine, readily distribute into the fetal circulation and may cause respiratory depression after birth. (9) For this reason, when obstetric analgesia is desired, meperidine (Demerol) should be administered within one hour of delivery. (10) The greatest degree of respiratory depression has been observed when the drug is given three to four hours before birth. (10)

Salicylates

Animal studies and retrospective human studies have suggested that salicylates (aspirin preparations) may be teratogenic. (11) However, the results of prospective human studies have been contradictory. (4) Data regarding decreased birth weight and increased perinatal mortality secondary to third trimester salicylate usage were also conflicting. (11) Nevertheless, aspirin-induced impaired hemostasis in both mother and neonate has been well documented and, as a result, it is best to avoid aspirin preparations during pregnancy. (12) Aspirin can also cause closure of the ductus arteriosus because it inhibits prostaglandin synthesis in the smooth muscle of the ductus.

Acetaminophen

Acetaminophen appears to be a relatively safe drug when taken in the usual therapeutic dose. Adverse effects resulting from its use during pregnancy have yet to be identified. (11)

Nonsteroidal-Antiinflammatory Drugs

Nonsteroidal-antiinflammatory drugs, when used during the third trimester, may produce an adverse effect on the fetus. These agents inhibit prostaglandin synthesis and may, therefore, stimulate closure of the ductus arteriosus in utero. (5) This would be accompanied by increased pulmonary artery pressure and difficulty in establishing pulmonary circulation after birth. (9) These drugs may also precipitate bleeding episodes via a platelet inhibitory effect, similar to that of aspirin. (5)

ANTIBIOTICS

Penicillins, Cephalosporins, and Erythromycin

Penicillins are safe to use in pregnancy. Although the safety of cephalosporins is not as well documented, there are no reports of teratogenicity associated with cephalosporin therapy. (13)

In patients allergic to penicillin, erythromycin may be safely used. (4)

Aminoglycosides

Aminoglycosides present a risk of fetal ototoxicity. Streptomycin has been demonstrated to cause toxicity to the fetal ear, and should be replaced by other agents when treating tuberculosis. (6) The fetal ototoxicity of gentamicin and tobramycin, although not as well documented as for streptomycin, necessitates that these drugs be used only for severe infections when no reasonable alternative exists. (4)

Antitubercular Drugs

Aside from streptomycin, other antitubercular agents (isoniazid, ethambutol, rifampcin) have not been shown to significantly increase the risk of birth defects. (14)

Tetracycline

Tetracycline readily crosses the placental barrier and gets deposited in fetal bones and teeth. (15) The exact effect of the drug on limb development is not well established, but discoloration of the teeth can occur if given to the prospective mother from the end of the first trimester throughout the remainder of pregnancy. (4, 6) Tetracyclines are clearly contraindicated during pregnancy.

Sulfonamides and Trimethoprim

Sulfonamides, although not specifically teratogenic, should be avoided during the latter weeks of pregnancy due to their tendency to displace bilirubin from plasma protein binding sites. (4) This effect may lead to neonatal jaundice and, possibly, kernicterus. (15)

Co-trimoxazole (sulfamethoxazole and trimethoprim) should also be avoided during the first trimester due to the possibility of causing birth defects which may arise from folate antagonism. (15)

Metronidazole

Metronidazole has not been shown to be teratogenic in humans. (4) However, animal studies have suggested potential carcinogenic and mutagenic properties. Generally, it is best to avoid using metronidazole during the first trimester. (15)

Chloramphenicol

Chloramphenicol crosses the placenta, but is not considered to be harmful to the fetus. Toxic effects were not demonstrated in newborns when up to 1 g was administered every 2 hours to women in labor. (16)

Lincomycin and Clindamycin

Lincomycin and clindamycin have not been shown to be teratogenic. (4, 17)

ANTICOAGULANTS

Warfarin administration during the first trimester causes a specific syndrome of fetal defects referred to as warfarin embryopathy or fetal warfarin syndrome. (18) Clinical manifestations include nasal hypoplasia, chondrodysplasia punctata, and possible mental retardation. (3) Second or third trimester exposure is more likely to be associated with central nervous system anomalies, including retardation, optic nerve atrophy, and microcephaly. (19) Warfarin therapy is also associated with hemorrhagic complications: mortality from perinatal hemorrhage is approximately 15%. (5)

Heparin is a large molecular-weight mucopolysaccharide which does not cross the placenta. (19) Despite the fact that heparin does not exert a direct effect on the fetus, its chronic administration is not without deleterious maternal effects, including hemorrhage, osteoporosis, and neurologic complications. (18)

Most authorities continue to recommend heparin as the anticoagulant drug of choice in pregnant women. (2, 15, 19-21) However, because heparin therapy itself is not without potentially serious complications, controversy regarding its usefulness remains, and some clinicians contend that warfarin is a reasonable therapeutic alternative. (18) Nevertheless, since mortality from antepartum thromboembolism is 15% for untreated patients compared to < 1% for treated patients, the main point to be made is that deep vein thrombosis during pregnancy should be treated, regardless of which drug is chosen. (2)

ANTICONVULSANTS

The risk of congenital malformations in an infant born to an
epileptic mother is estimated to be two to three times greater
than that of the general population. (22) The most common abnormalities include cleft palate, cardiac anomalies, and minor
skeletal defects. Aside from drug usage, other potential teratogenic risk factors, such as the occurrence of seizures during
pregnancy, should also be considered. Therefore, continued
antiepileptic treatment of the mother is desirable. Indeed, studies designed to evaluate the teratogenicity of anticonvulsant
drugs generally use nonepileptic women for the control group. (5)

Seizure Therapy

The primary concern in treating a pregnant epileptic patient
should be to maintain an effective seizure control. Of course,
if the woman has been seizure-free for years, a trial of gradual
medication withdrawal may be indicated. (23) One should note,
however, that even if phenytoin therapy is required to maintain
effective seizure control, the patient still has a 90% chance of
giving birth to a normal child. (24)

Birth defects are not the only concern related to fetal well-
being in the pregnant epileptic patient; additional complications
in the neonate have been associated with maternal anticonvulsant therapy. A withdrawal syndrome, manifested by hyperex-
citability, tremor, and restlessness, has been observed in the
newborns of mothers who took phenobarbital, 60-120 mg/day,
during the last trimester. (22) Furthermore, neonates exposed
to phenytoin, barbiturates, or trimethadione in utero may develop bleeding tendencies during the first 24 hours postpartum
due to a deficiency of vitamin K-dependent clotting factors. (9)

Phenytoin

The fetal hydantoin syndrome, characterized by craniofacial
anomalies, limb defects, deficient growth, and mental retardation, is the most commonly reported syndrome associated with
a specific anticonvulsant agent. (22) Approximately 7-11% of
children exposed to phenytoin in utero display the fetal hydantoin
syndrome. (24)

Trimethadione, Phenobarbital, Primidone

The causal relationship between exposure and teratogenesis is better established for trimethadione than for any other anticonvulsant drug. Clinical characteristics of the hydantoin and trimethadione syndromes are quite similar; in fact, similar birth defects have also been associated with in utero exposure to phenobarbital or primidone. (22)

Carbamazepine

Carbamazepine has not, to date, been implicated as a teratogenic agent. (4, 22)

Valproic Acid

Animal studies have shown a variety of teratogenic effects of this new anticonvulsant drug, yet case reports of valproic acid-induced human dysmorphogenesis have been extremely rare. (25) Recent evidence, however, suggests a link between first trimester valproic acid use and an increased risk of spina bifida. (26)

ANTIEMETICS

No definitive association has been established between antiemetic therapy and congenital malformations. When used judiciously, agents such as promethazine, prochlorperazine, diphenhydrinate, or a combination of doxylamine/pyridoxine represent a safe form of therapy for nausea during pregnancy. (15, 27)

The combination product of doxylamine/pyridoxine (Bendectin) has recently been implicated as a possible teratogen, thus causing alarm over its widespread use among pregnant women. However, two large-scale studies failed to demonstrate a cause-effect relationship between Bendectin and birth defects. (28, 29) Bendectin was recently withdrawn from the U.S. market by its manufacturer.

ANTINEOPLASTIC DRUGS

Cytotoxic agents constitute a particular risk to the fetus during the first trimester, a period of rapid cell division and organogenesis. (3) The greatest risk of fetal malformation has been associated with methotrexate, a folic acid antagonist. (2) Methotrexate-induced fetal abnormalities, including hydrocephulus, cleft palate, and meningomyelocele, occur at an incidence exceeding 50%. (30)

Antineoplastic therapy should be avoided during the first trimester of pregnancy unless absolutely necessary, and every effort should be made to refrain from using methotrexate. Beyond the first trimester, the administration of cytotoxic drugs does not appear to increase the likelihood of congenital abnormalities. (30) However, one must always consider the possibility of long-term consequences resulting from exposure to cytotoxic drugs in utero. (2)

CARDIOVASCULAR DRUGS

Diuretics

Diuretics should generally be avoided during pregnancy. Thiazides have caused maternal electrolyte imbalances, hyperglycemia, hyperuricemia, and pancreatitis. (19) Neonatal complications at birth include hypoglycemia, hyperbilirubinemia, thrombocytopenia, and hemolysis. (31) Although no specific toxic or teratogenic effects have been noted with furosemide therapy, it may cause metabolic complications in the pregnant patient.

As a rule, diuretics should be reserved for cases of severe left ventricular failure or severe hypertension not responsive to a single antihypertensive agent. (19, 31) Should diuretic therapy be warranted, furosemide appears to be the agent of choice, (19) but every precaution should be taken to guard against electrolytic and metabolic complications.

Antihypertensives

Of all the antihypertensive drugs currently available, reserpine is the only one to have been implicated as being a teratogen, and is clearly contraindicated during pregnancy. (19)

Methyldopa and hydralazine have been used extensively in treating hypertension in pregnancy. Both drugs have been shown to be safe and effective. (20, 32)

Reports have indicated that beta-blockers may cause adverse fetal effects, including bradycardia, hypoglycemia, neonatal respiratory distress, and intrauterine growth retardation. (5) However, to date, no beta-blocker has been shown to be teratogenic, and the clinical significance of the aforementioned fetal effects is highly controversial. Beta-blockers do not currently represent the drug of choice for treatment of hypertension in pregnancy, although further investigation is warranted. (19, 33)

Clonidine does not produce adverse fetal effects and may be used in pregnancy, yet it appears to offer little, if any, advantage over methyldopa. (20, 32)

In treating hypertensive emergencies during pregnancy, hydralazine seems to be the agent of choice, although diazoxide may represent a reasonable alternative. (34) Nitroprusside may also play a role, but further human studies are needed before it can be recommended routinely. (34)

Cardiac Glycosides and Antiarrhythmic Drugs

Digoxin and digitoxin have not been shown to be teratogenic in humans. (19) Palpitation, paroxysmal atrial tachycardia and premature ventricular beats are often observed during pregnancy, especially because recent improvements in medical or surgical management of patients with cardiac and valvular disease make it possible for such patients to become pregnant. Lidocaine, quinidine, procainamide, disopyramide, and beta blockers are relatively safe in controlling such arrhythmias provided the usual caution in the use of antiarrhythmic drugs is exercised. Only limited data are available on the clinical usefulness of verapamil during pregnancy, but this new calcium channel blocker appears to be safe in such patients for effective control of maternal as well as fetal arrhythmias.

HORMONES

Estrogens

Diethylstilbestrol (DES) has been definitively linked to the development of vaginal adenocarcinoma in the female progeny of women who took the drug during pregnancy. (3) The onset of this tumor occurs between 7 and 29 years of age. The risk of clear cell adenocarcinoma of the vagina or cervix in DES-exposed females up to age 24 appears to range from 0.14 to 1.4 per 1000. (35) DES-exposed males have demonstrated hypotrophic testes, epididymal cysts, and a 32% incidence of abnormal spermatozoal analyses. (3)

Clomiphene is the only other estrogenic compound to have been implicated as a teratogen. Chromosomal abnormalities such as trisomy 21 and aneuploidy have been observed in offspring and aborted fetuses of women who conceived following induced ovulation. (3)

Progestins/Androgens

Intrauterine exposure to progestins or androgens has resulted in masculinization of female genitalia of the offspring. (35) These changes have been most commonly reported with norethindrone or ethisterone therapy. Some studies suggest an increased risk of congenital anomalies among offspring of women who were taking oral contraceptives at the time of conception. (2) These abnormalities are described as the VACTREL syndrome (vertebral, anal, cardiac, tracheal, renal, esophageal, limb), although evidence of the cause-effect relationship is not conclusive. (35)

PSYCHOTROPIC DRUGS

Anxiolytics/Sedative-Hypnotics

Studies have indicated that there may be an increased risk of cleft lip or cleft palate in infants exposed to diazepam during the first trimester of pregnancy. (3) Chlordiazepoxide exposure during the first 42 days of pregnancy may also increase the incidence of central nervous system abnormalities. (9)

One should also consider that chronic use of a benzodiazepine as a class of drugs throughout pregnancy may precipitate withdrawal symptoms in the newborn. (15) An additional concern is that drugs such as diazepam, which are slowly metabolized by the neonate, may persist in the fetal circulation for an extended period of time after birth. On theoretical grounds at least, if a benzodiazepine is indicated shortly before delivery, a drug which is more easily metabolized, such as lorazepam or oxazepam, might be preferable. (5) Certainly, these drugs may be better tolerated by both the mother and the neonate than the barbiturate group of drugs.

Antidepressants

Tricyclic antidepressants should be avoided, especially during the first trimester of pregnancy, due to reports suggesting the likelihood of teratogenicity. (15) When administered later in pregnancy, neonates may manifest signs of tricyclic toxicity, including tachycardia and irritability.

Antipsychotics

Data regarding an association between congenital cardiovascular malformations and phenothiazine exposure during the first trimester of pregnancy are conflicting. (3) Infants born to mothers who have been on long-term phenothiazine therapy may manifest extrapyramidal signs, which begin within 24 hours after birth and persist, if untreated, for up to nine months. (9) Short-term use of a phenothiazine prior to delivery for control of nausea or to potentiate analgesia may be accomplished without any adverse effect on the newborn.

Lithium

Lithium is contraindicated during the first trimester of pregnancy due to an increased incidence of congenital heart disease. (2) Maternal lithium therapy may also affect the thyroid function of the fetus or mother. (9) Therapy during the last trimester may produce metabolic complications in the neonate, due to slow lithium elimination after birth. (36)

SOCIAL DRUGS

Smoking

Maternal smoking has been associated with intrauterine growth retardation, spontaneous abortion, prematurity, still-birth, abruptio placenta, and premature rupture of the membranes. (9, 37) The perinatal death risk appears to be somewhat related to the quantity of cigarettes smoked: 20% for smokers of less than one pack per day and 35% for those who smoke more than one pack per day. (9)

The influence of maternal smoking on the incidence of congenital malformations is not well defined. (3)

Alcohol

Fetal alcohol syndrome, a dysmorphic condition characterized by facial anomalies, growth deficiencies, and central nervous system dysfunction, was first described in 1968. (38) One prospective study involving 633 women indicated that the incidence of congenital abnormalities in infants born to heavy drinkers (more than 45 ml absolute alcohol per day) may be as high as 32%. (39) Generally, the risk of fetal alcohol syndrome is low if the average alcohol ingestion remains below one ounce per day of absolute alcohol, (40) though complete abstinence would be preferable.

Caffeine

Although a definite cause-effect relationship has not been established, one retrospective study demonstrated that pregnant women who consume more than 600 mg of caffeine per day have a higher incidence of abortion and prematurity. (9)

Drugs of Abuse

The teratogenicity of marijuana has not been defined. (3) However, since marijuana may cause chromosomal damage, a direct effect on the fetus cannot be ruled out. (41)

The fetus may become addicted to a narcotic in utero, and may, in turn, develop a withdrawal syndrome of irritability, tremor, tachypnea, restlessness, convulsions, and a "high pitch" cry after birth. (5) Maternal narcotic addiction may also lead to such obstetric complications as premature labor, breech delivery, toxemia, and low birth weight. (3) After birth, the physical and mental development of the infant also may be impaired. (5)

The incidence of neonatal withdrawal is reduced and the overall outcome of pregnancy is enhanced when the narcotic-addicted pregnant patients are placed on low-dose methadone maintenance therapy. (5, 42)

MISCELLANEOUS DRUGS

Vaccines(43)

As a general rule, live, attenuated-virus vaccines (rubella, measles, mumps) are contraindicated in pregnant women. However, yellow fever and oral polio vaccine can be given to pregnant women who are at high risk of exposure to natural infection. In this circumstance, it is best to delay the vaccine until the second or third trimester of pregnancy.

There is no evidence of risk to the fetus from maternal immunization using inactivated virus vaccines, bacterial vaccines, toxoids, or immune globulin.

Corticosteroids

Corticosteroids appear to present very little risk to the fetus. Extensive use of corticosteroids in pregnant women has failed to identify an associated increase in malformation, growth retardation, premature labor, or adrenocortical insufficiency. (44) The short-term use of betamethasone to prevent respiratory

distress syndrome in premature neonates transiently reduces
cord blood cortisol concentration in the cord blood but does not
impair the infant's cortisol response to stress. (5) The benefits
of betamethasone administration for prevention of respiratory
distress syndrome clearly outweigh the potential risk of neonatal infection. (44)

Antithyroid Drugs

Propylthiouracil and methimazole may cause an infant to be
goitrous at birth. (9) The maternal fetal serum level ratio of
propylthiouracil is lower than that of methimazole, but the
clinical significance of this observation is unknown. (40)

The fetal thyroid begins to concentrate iodine after the 14th
week of gestation. (5) Consequently, the administration of radioactive iodine (^{131}I or ^{125}I) after the first trimester of pregnancy
is contraindicated. (9, 45) One should also avoid potassium iodide,
a common ingredient in many over-the-counter cough and cold
preparations. (5)

Oral Hypoglycemics

Despite isolated case reports, oral hypoglycemic drugs
(sulfonylureas) have not proven to be teratogenic. However,
since these agents can cross the placenta and stimulate fetal
insulin release, they should probably be discontinued at least
48 hours prior to delivery to avoid neonatal hypoglycemia. (4)

Isotretinoin

Isotretinoin (Accutane) is a vitamin A analog recently ap-
proved for treatment of severe recalcitrant cystic acne. Definite teratogenicity has been observed in animals and in humans
given isotretinoin and this drug is contraindicated during pregnancy. Physicians contemplating using isotretinoin in women
of childbearing potential should prescribe an effective form of
contraception before therapy is started. They should also discuss the desirability of continuation of pregnancy if the patient
becomes pregnant while receiving isotretinoin.

DRUGS AND BREAST FEEDING

After birth, the concerns regarding a mother's drug therapy
adversely affecting her child are not necessarily eliminated.
Certainly, should the mother decide to breast feed, the potential
for drug transfer from mother to child persists. Various factors

relating to the mother, the child, and the specific drug in question determine the extent to which the drug is able to exert a pharmacologic effect on the newborn infant. These multiple factors must be considered when evaluating the drug therapy of a breast-feeding patient.

Physicochemical Factor

The total amount of drug that diffuses into breast milk is increased for drugs which are less protein bound; whereas drugs which are more lipid soluble diffuse at a higher rate. Since the pH of milk (6.8-7.3) is less than that of plasma (7.4), weak bases tend to exist in a more ionized state (and are thus "trapped") in milk; the opposite is true for weak acid.(46)

Pharmacokinetic Factors

The plasma-concentrations of a drug fluctuate between high (peak) and low (trough) levels during intermittent drug dosing. Since passage into breast milk occurs primarily via passive diffusion, the maximum milk concentration which can be achieved in the breast milk depends upon the equilibrium established between unbound drug in the milk and plasma. Obviously, a drug which diffuses into milk slowly in relation to its overall serum elimination rate will most likely achieve a low milk concentration. (47)

In this regard, drug transfer into breast milk would be greater during long-term chronic dosing than after short-term acute administration, due to the establishment of steady-state serum levels with chronic therapy. (48)

In general, drugs with an overall smaller volume of distribution produce higher serum levels, thereby resulting in higher levels in the breast milk. (49)

Maternal and Infant Factors

Along with the magnitude of the dose prescribed, the relationship between the time of drug administration and breast-feeding times represents another important therapeutic consideration. Generally, nursing the infant immediately before the administration of a dose will result in the lowest possible concentration of drug in the milk at the next feeding. (48)

In assessing the potential effect of the drug on the infant, one should also consider the relative quantity of milk consumed by the infant, the extent of drug transfer into breast milk, the potential toxicity of the drug, and the oral bioavailability of the drug in the infant. (47, 50)

Guidelines for Use of Drugs in Breast-Feeding Mothers (47, 50, 51)

1. If a drug is given as a single daily dose, administer just prior to the infant's longest sleep period.

2. If a drug is give in multiple daily doses, schedule feeding times to avoid peak drug levels.

3. If a short course of therapy with a toxic drug is required, temporarily discontinue breast feeding.

4. When in doubt as to the amount of drug in the breast milk, measure the concentration.

5. The amount of drug in human milk is rarely greater than 1-2% of the maternal dose. This amount is usually not hazardous to the infant. Nursing should only be interrupted for a few, highly toxic drugs such as lithium, cytotoxic drugs (cyclophosphamide), antimetabolities, radioactive pharmaceuticals, phenindione, chloramphenicol, and isoniazid. (48-50)

Refer to Tables 11-1, 11-2, and 11-3 for further information on drugs that may adversely affect the mother or fetus.

Table 11-1: Adverse effects of maternal drugs on the fetus or neonate.

Drugs	First Trimester	Third Trimester	Comments
ANALGESICS			
Acetaminophen	0	0	
Nonsteroidal-Anti-inflammatory drugs	0	+++	Premature closure of ductus arteriosus
Narcotics	0	+++	Respiratory depression, neonatal withdrawal syndrome
Salicylates	+	+++	Neonatal bleeding tendency
ANTIBIOTICS			
Aminoglycosides	++	++	Ototoxicity, avoid streptomycin
Cephalosporins	0	0	
Chloramphenicol	0	0	

Table 11-1 (continued)

Drugs	First Trimester	Third Trimester	Comments
SOCIAL DRUGS			
Alcohol	+++	+++	Fetal alcohol syndrome; "safe" intake level unknown
Caffeine	+	+	Increased risk of spontaneous abortion with large intake (7600 mg/day)
Smoking	++	++	Intrauterine growth retardation
MISCELLANEOUS DRUGS			
Antihistamines	0	0	
Antithyroids	+	+	Reversible neonatal hypothyroidism
Corticosteroids	0	0	Consider maternal effects
General anesthetics (short-term exposure)	0	0	
Sulfonamides	0	+++	Neonatal jaundice

Clindamycin	0	0	
Erythromycin base	0	0	
Ethambutol	0	0	
Isoniazid	0	0	
Metronidazole	+	0	Possible carcinogenesis or mutagenesis
Penicillins	0	0	
Rifampin	0	0	
Tetracyclines	+++	+++	Contraindicated
Trimethoprim	+	0	Folate antagonist, avoid during first trimester
ANTICOAGULANTS			
Heparin	0	0	Consider maternal effects
Warfarin	+++	+++	Fetal warfarin syndrome; contraindicated

Table 11-1 (continued)

Drugs	First Trimester	Third Trimester	Comments
ANTICONVULSANTS			
Carbamazepine	0	0	
Phenobarbital (and Primidone)	++	++	Possible teratogenicity; neonatal withdrawal syndrome
Phenytoin	+++	+	Fetal hydantoin syndrome
Trimethadione	+++	+	Most teratogenic anticonvulsant
Valproic acid	+	0	Possible spina bifida
ANTINEOPLASTICS			
Alkylating agents	+	0	Especially busulfan and cyclophosphamide: avoid combination therapy
Antimetabolites	+++	0	Avoid methotrexate during first trimester

CARDIOVASCULAR DRUGS

Drug			Comments
Diuretics	0	0	Consider maternal effects
Antihypertensives			
Beta blockers	+	+	Possible intrauterine growth retardation; neonatal bradycardia and hypoglycemia
Clonidine	0	0	
Hydralazine	0	0	
Methyldopa	0	0	Drug of choice
Reserpine	+	+	Possible teratogenicity; neonatal nasal stuffiness
Antiarrhythmics			
Digoxin	0	0	
Disopyramide	0	0	Limited data available
Lidocaine	0	0	Toxicity may occur if administered during fetal acidosis

Table 11-1 (continued)

Drugs	First Trimester	Third Trimester	Comments
Procainamide	0	0	Consider possible SLE
Quinidine	0	0	
Verapamil	0	0	Limited data available
HORMONES			
DES	+++	++	Contraindicated; carcinogenic in females; testicular abnormalities in males
Clomiphene	+	+	Possible trisomy 21
Progestins/Androgens	+++	+++	Contraindicated; masculinization of females
Inorganic iodides	+++	++	Avoid
Oral hypoglycemics	+	++	Neonatal hypoglycemia

Radioactive iodine	+++	+++	Contraindicated
Theophylline	0	+	Transient neonatal tachycardia
Thyroid hormone	0	0	
PSYCHOTROPIC DRUGS			
Amphetamines	+	+	Possible teratogenicity; avoid
Benzodiazepines	+	+	Possible teratogenicity; neonatal withdrawal
Haloperidol	+	+	Possible neonatal extrapyramidal symptoms
Lithium	+++	+	Congenital cardiac defects; contraindicated first trimester
Phenothiazines	+	+	Short-term antiemetic use okay
Tricyclic antidepressants	+	+	Possible teratogenicity; neonatal withdrawal syndrome

Table 11-1 (continued)

Drugs	First Trimester	Third Trimester	Comments
Vaccines			
Attenuated virus	++	+	Contraindicated first trimester
Bacterial	0	0	
Immune globulin	0	0	
Killed virus	0	0	
Toxoids	0	0	
Vitamin A analogues (Isotretinoin)	+++	+++	Contraindicated

+++   Well established cause-effect relationship
++   Probable cause-effect relationship
+   Possible cause-effect relationship
0   No cause-effect relationship documented, probably safe to use
Note: All drugs should be avoided during pregnancy whenever possible.

Table 11-2: Drugs to be used with caution by lactating women.

Drug	Adverse Effect on Infant
Alcohol	Large consumption may intoxicate infant
Amantadine	May cause vomiting, rash, urinary retention
Amphetamines	May cause irritability, insomnia
Antineoplastic drugs	Limited data; best to avoid
Barbiturates	May cause drowsiness; short-acting preferable to long-acting
Caffeine	Large intake may cause irritability
Diuretics	May suppress lactation or cause maternal dehydration
Metronidazole	May cause anorexia, vomiting (don't breast feed for 12-14 hours after 2 gram dose)
Non-steroidal anti-inflammatory drugs	Unknown effects; use with caution
Penicillins/ Cephalosporins	Only small quantities absorbed, but could be enough to cause allergic sensitization
Radiopharmaceuticals	Do not breast feed while radioactive material is in breast milk Time required for elimination: Gallium-69: 2 weeks Iodine-125: 12 days Iodine-131: 7-10 days Technetium-99: 2 days
Salicylates	May cause bleeding tendency

Table 11-2 (continued)

Drug	Adverse Effect on Infant
Sulfonamides	May cause jaundice in neonate; avoid in G-6-PD deficient infant
Tetracyclines	May cause teeth mottling, but due to Ca^{++} binding in milk, little drug is absorbed by infant
Vitamin D	High doses may cause hypercalcemia

Table 11-3: Drugs which should be avoided by lactating women.

Drug	Adverse Effect on Infant
Benzodiazepines	Lethargy
Bromocriptine	(Suppresses lactation)
Chloramphenicol	Bone marrow suppression
Cimetidine	CNS stimulation
Clemastine	**Drowsiness**, irritability
Cyclophosphamide	Immune suppression
Ergotamine	Vomiting, diarrhea, convulsions
Gold salts	Rash, liver and kidney inflammation
Iodides	Thyroid suppression
Isoniazid	Possible hepatotoxicity
Lithium	CNS effects of lithium toxicity (infant blood level reaches 30-50% of maternal blood level)
Methimazole	Interference with thyroid function
Phenindione (warfarin is okay)	Hemorrhage
Propylthiouracil	Decreased thyroid function
Reserpine	Nasal stuffiness
Vitamin A analogues (Isotretinoin)	Limited data available: best to avoid

REFERENCES

1. Shepard, TH. Detection of human teratogenic agents. J. Pediatr., 101(5):810, 1982.

2. Beeley, L. Adverse effects of drugs in the first trimester of pregnancy. Clin. Obstet. Gynecol., 8(2):261, 1981.

3. Golbus, MS. Teratology for the obstetrician: Current status. Obstet. Gynecol., 55(3):269, 1980.

4. Hays, DP. Teratogenesis: A review of the basic principles with a discussion of selected agents: Part II. Drug Intell. Clin. Pharm., 15:542, 1981.

5. Beeley, L. Adverse effects of drugs in later pregnancy. Clin. Obstet. Gynecol., 8(2):275, 1981.

6. Levy, G. Pharmacokinetics of fetal and neonatal exposure to drugs. Obstet. Gynecol., 58(5):95, 1981.

7. Anon. Pregnancy labeling. FDA Drug Bull., 9(4):23, 1979.

8. Anon. Pregnancy categories for prescription drugs. FDA Bull., 12(3):24, 1982.

9. Hill, RM, and Stern, L. Drugs in pregnancy: effects on the fetus and newborn. Drugs, 17:182, 1979.

10. Ricciarelli, EA, Gursche, BB, and Smith, TC. Opioids and obstetrics. Clin. Obstet. Gynecol., 17(2):259, 1974.

11. Collins, E. Maternal and fetal effects of acetaminophen and salicylates in pregnancy. Obstet. Gynecol., 58(5):575, 1981.

12. Stuart, MJ, Gross, JJ, Elrod, H, et al. Effects of acetyl-salicyclic-acid ingestion on maternal and neonatal hemostasis. N. Engl. J. Med., 307(15):909, 1982.

13. Ledger, WJ. Antibiotics in pregnancy. Clin. Obstet. Gynecol., 20(2):411, 1977.

14. Scheinhorn, DJ, and Angelillo, VA. Antituberculous therapy in pregnancy. West. J. Med., 127:195, 1977.

15. Rao, JM, and Arulappu, R. Drug use in pregnancy: How to avoid problems. Drugs, 22:409, 1981.

16. Weinstein, AJ. Treatment of bacterial infections in pregnancy. Drugs, 17:56, 1979.

17. Hays, DP. Teratogenesis: A review of the basic principles with a discussion of selected agents: Part I. Drug Intell. Clin. Pharm., 15:444, 1981.

18. Hall, JG, Pauli, RM, and Wilson, KM. Maternal and fetal sequelae of anticoagulation during pregnancy. Am. J. Med., 68:122, 1980.

19. Witter, FR, King, TM, and Blake, DA. Adverse effects of cardiovascular drug therapy on the fetus and neonate. Obstet. Gynecol., 58(5):1005, 1981.

20. Waters, WA, and Humphrey, MD. Common medical disorders in pregnancy and their treatment. Drugs, 19:455, 1980.

21. Tawes, RL, Kennedy, PA, and Harris, EJ, et al. Management of deep venous thrombosis and pulmonary embolism during pregnancy. Am. J. Surg., 144:141, 1982.

22. Montouris, GD, Fenichel, GM, and McLain, LW. The pregnant epileptic: A review and recommendations. Arch. Neurol., 36:601, 1979.

23. Hanson, JW, and Buehler, BA. Fetal hydantoin syndrome: Current status. J. Pediatr., 101(5):816, 1982.

24. Committee on Drugs. Valproic acid: Benefits and risks. Pediatrics, 70(2):316, 1982.

25. Anon. Valproic acid and spina bifida: A preliminary report - France. MMWR, 31(42):565, 1982.

26. Committee on drugs. Anticonvulsants and pregnancy. Pediatrics, 63(2):331, 1980.

27. Witter, FR, King, TM, and Blake, DA: The effects of chronic gastrointestinal medication on the fetus and neonate. Obstet. Gynecol., 58(5):795, 1981.

28. Cordero, JF, Oakley, GP, and Greenberg, F, et al. Is bendectin a teratogen? JAMA, 245(22):2307, 1981.

29. Mitchell, AA, Rosenberg, L, and Shapiro, S, et al. Birth defects related to bendectin use in pregnancy. JAMA, 245(22):2311, 1981.

30. Barber, HR. Fetal and neonatal effects of cytotoxic agents. Obstet. Gynecol., 58(5):415, 1981.

31. Redman, CW. Treatment of hypertension in pregnancy. Kidney Int., 18:267, 1980.

32. Redman, CW. The use of antihypertensive drugs in hypertension in pregnancy. Clin. Obstet. Gynecol., 4(3):685, 1977.

33. Rubin, PC. Beta blockers in pregnancy. N. Engl. J. Med., 305(23):1323, 1981.

34. Nissen, JC. Treatment of hypertensive emergencies of pregnancy. Clin. Pharm., 1:334, 1982.

35. Herbst, AL. Diethylstilbestrol and other sex hormones during pregnancy. Obstet. Gynecol., 58(5):355, 1981.

36. Sriwatanakul, K, and Weis, O. Using antipsychotic drugs during pregnancy. Drug Ther. (Hosp.), 7(11):107, 1982.

37. Kline, J, Stein, ZA, Susser, M, et al. Smoking: A risk factor for spontaneous abortion. N. Engl. J. Med., 297(15):793, 1977.

38. Clarren, SK, and Smith, DW. The fetal alcohol syndrome. N. Engl. J. Med., 298(19):1063, 1978.

39. Ouellete, EM, Rosett, HL, and Rosman, NP, et al. Adverse effects on offspring of maternal alcohol abuse during pregnancy. N. Engl. J. Med., 297(10):528, 1977.

40. O'Brien, TE, and Balmer, JA. Drugs and the human fetus. US Pharm., 6(3):44, 1981.

41. Stenchever, MA, Kunysz, TJ, and Allen, MA. Chromosome breakage in users of marijuana. Am. J. Obstet. Gynecol., 118(1):106, 1974.

42. Blinick, G, Jerez, E, and Wallach, RC. Methadone maintenance, pregnancy, and progeny. JAMA, 225(5):477, 1973.

43. Anon. General recommendations on immunization. MMWR, 32(1):1, 1983.

44. Sidhu, RK, and Hawkins, DF. Corticosteroids. Clin. Obstet. Gynecol., 8(2):383, 1981.

45. Hays, DP. Teratogenesis: A review of the basic principles with a discussion of selected agents: Part III. Drug Intell. Clin. Pharm., 15:639, 1981.

46. Gaginella, TS. Drugs and the nursing mother-infant. US Pharm., 3(3):40, 1978.

47. Anderson, PO. Drugs and breast feeding. Sem. Perinat., 3(3):271, 1979.

48. Bowes, WA. The effect of medications on the lactating mother and her infant. Clin. Obstet. Gynecol., 23(4):1073, 1980.

49. Beeley, L. Drugs and breast feeding. Clin. Obstet. Gynecol., 8(2):291, 1981.

50. Berlin, CM. Pharmacologic considerations of drug abuse in the lactating mother. Obstet. Gynecol., 58(5):175, 1981.

51. Committee on Drugs. The transfer of drugs and other chemicals into human breast milk. Pediatrics, 72(3):375, 1983.

Chapter 12

OBSTETRICAL ADVANCES IN RELATION
TO SURGICAL PRACTICE

John L. Duhring, M.D.

During the last ten years dramatic progress has been made
in the diagnosis and treatment of pregnancy problems encountered coexistent with a surgical emergency. Until recently, the
trauma to the uterus from abdominal manipulation during surgery for other nongenital areas often resulted in premature labor and delivery. At that time the only things available to stop
premature labor were sedatives and analgesics, particularly
narcotics. The FDA release of beta mimetic agents such as
Terbutiline or Ritodrine have enabled effective tocolysis to result. These are beta mimetic drugs which decrease the sensitivity of the myeometrium to labor-inducing stimuli. They are
initially used intravenously and then, when control has been obtained, the patient is maintained on oral medication for at least
four weeks following the abdominal surgical procedure. These
drugs often have many troublesome side effects, although none
are serious. Some of the side effects are rapid pulse rate, a
decrease in serum potassium, increase in blood sugar, and
feelings of apprehension and anxiety. One should be very careful in treating hypokalemia with intravenous potassium because
actually the potassium has been moved from the vascular compartment into the intracellular compartment and there is not a
deficiency of potassium. Prior to the administration of supplemental amounts of potassium, one should always do an electro-
cardiogram to see if there really is a hypokalemic effect.
     Many inflammatory diseases such as ulcerative colitis will
require adrenal corticosteroids such as cortisone or prednisone
to arrest the inflammatory process. At one time, it was thought
these agents were capable of causing congenital malformations.
It is now apparent that these agents can safely be used in pregnancy and, although they do result in cleft lip and cleft palate

in animal species, such things have never been observed in humans on maintenance doses of cortisone.

Another interesting change in obstetrics and gynecology has been the marked decline in the number of cases of nausea and vomiting in pregnancy. It is very rare to see hyperemesis gravidarum at this time; 99.9% of the management of nausea and vomiting in pregnancy is diet. Rarely, if ever, is it necessary to depend upon drug usage to alleviate this situation. A bland diet with small, frequent feeding (6 per day) is advised. Certain foods, such as milk, citrus fruit juices, and highly spiced foods, are also prohibited under this diet plan.

The proliferation of new and more broad spectrum antibiotics has dramatically changed the therapy of intra-abdominal infection coexisting with pregnancy. The things to be remembered are that Chloromycetin can produce the Gray syndrome in a newborn and, therefore, chloramphenicol should be used with great care. Tetracycline derivatives, including the second and third generation offshoot, should not be used because these will stain the enamel of teeth as well as produce changes in growth of the bone. Cephalosporins, penicillin, and aminoglycosides are well-tolerated in pregnancy and, where indication exists for significant antibiotic treatment, these agents should be used with freedom. The most difficult patient to treat is one who is pregnant and has an allergy to penicillin and its derivatives. In these difficult cases, consultation should also be sought with an infectious disease specialist so that a program of management specifically tailored for the infection and the particular patient is always obtained.

Developments in **anesthesia** have really opened more questions than they give answers. It used to be said that general anesthesia should be avoided for the pregnant patient because of problems of oxygenation. With the new inhalatory anesthetic agents, oxygenation should never be a problem and, if an oxygen concentration of at least 20% in the inspired areas is obtained, there will be no problem with the baby. Certainly, the use of conduction anesthesia, either epidural or spinal, does not cause a problem either. This is provided the patient is tilted to the right or left side by a hip roll, so that the pregnant uterus does not fall back on the vena cava and eclude it with relaxation of the abdominal muscles by the blocking anesthesia. There is very little to choose between these. Both spinal anesthesia and general anesthesia have assets as well as liabilities. It probably has been said that the best anesthetic to use for a pregnant woman requiring surgery is the agent or technique most familiar to the anesthesiologist. Whatever he feels he is comfortable with and better able to control the patient with is probably the best choice to arrive at.

Hyperalimentation has become a very valuable part of obstetrical practice. Patients with severe nausea and vomiting in pregnancy (hyperemesis gravidarum) are often effectively treated by subclavian line, allowing intravenous hyperalimentation. This should be carried on at an appropriate rate so as to avoid acidosis because at least one study seems to indicate that starvation ketoacidosis may have a deleterious effect on the brain growth and development of a fetus. A study, published in 1969 by Churchill, recommends that all attempts should be made to avoid starvation acidosis.

The development of the electronic fetal monitor has greatly altered the approach to surgical procedures. With the external devices being as precise and accurate as they are, one can follow the status of the fetus in utero both pre- and postoperatively for other nonpelvic surgeries. The use of the electronic fetal monitor will allow one to diagnose and institute appropriate corrective measures if fetal distress is encountered.

The use of ultrasound in obstetrics has greatly increased the diagnostic accuracy of the clinician. This test is particularly useful in the patient with lower abdominal pain where the pregnancy test on the blood has been positive and one is dealing with a question of appendicitis vs ectopic pregnancy vs intrauterine pregnancy. In these cases ultrasound will certainly enable one to see and diagnose an intrauterine fetus, and this would effectively rule out the possibility of ectopic pregnancy. Ultrasound has also been found very useful in measuring the gestational age of the fetus and in enabling safe amniotic fluid biopsies to be performed for either genetic or maturity reasons. At the present time, genetic abnormalities can be excluded by doing an amniocentesis at roughly the 16th week of pregnancy and growing the fetal cells in tissue culture. An extra chromosome or the deletion of a chromosome may indicate fetal development problems that may, in certain circumstances, warrant consideration of pregnancy termination. The other use for ultrasound and amniocentesis is at the end of pregnancy when one is attempting to define the maturity of the baby. This is done by obtaining a specimen of amniotic fluid by amniocentesis and analyzing it for one of four tests:

1. amniotic fluid fat cells
2. amniotic fluid bilirubinoid pigments
3. amniotic fluid creatinine
4. amniotic LSH ratio with phosphotidal glycerol added

By using one or more of these tests one can very precisely evaluate the baby in terms of extrauterine existence. If the amniotic fluid shows an immature fetus, then, if at all possible, it would be better to wait until some later time for delivery. However, if delivery must be accomplished for other reasons, then at least the neonatal staff can be alerted to the fact that it will not only have a premature baby, but a premature baby with immature lungs, and it may anticipate respiratory problems. Ultrasound is also extremely useful in vaginal bleeding during pregnancy, where the question is always whether the problem is 1) a placenta previa, 2) abruptio placenta, or 3) even more unusual in that there is a local factor, such as a cervical laceration, which accounts for the bleeding. Ultrasound will allow one to precisely localize the placenta, and therein negate the possibility of placenta previa. Also, in many cases it is possible to see the retroplacental clot, and sometimes it is possible to diagnose abruptio placenta. Once these uterine factors have been excluded as possible sites of bleeding, then a careful, gentle pelvic examination may reveal a lower genital tract site for the bleeding.

Diagnostic x rays have for many years received a bad name in obstetrical patients. The fact of the matter is that it takes 50-100 rad to cause significant malformation. This must be delivered at a critical time in pregnancy (i.e., 6-8 weeks). In doing the total abdominal work-up — including an upper and lower gastrointestinal series, a cholecystogram, and intravenous pyelogram — only about 1 rad is delivered to the fetus from these multiple diagnostic procedures. Therefore, we are well within the margin of safety and obviously we are not advocating the prophylactic use of x rays for any reason. However, if there is a valid indication for x rays, then one should proceed with due caution, recognizing that the baby is there but probably will not be harmed. Unfortunately, some nonobstetrical physicians encountering a menstruating woman with an abdominal problem will rush ahead and get a full battery of x-rays and then, when they discover the patient is pregnant, it is almost a reflex to suggest pregnancy termination. This is obviously not necessary in most cases and can be done on an elective basis if the patient feels that she would not want to take any chance at all with the well-being of her baby.

While the venogram remains the standard for the diagnosis of deep thrombophlebitis, many physicians have now turned to very effective use of Doppler ultrasound to diagnose an occlusion of the deep femoral vessels.

In summary, the woman who is pregnant and has a coexisting surgical disease must be treated pretty much the same as her nonpregnant sister would be. There are certain drugs which should not be used, such as the Warfarin compounds, chloramphenicol, tetracycline derivatives, and sulfa drugs. X-ray studies should not electively be ordered on anyone, but if x rays are necessary to make a diagnosis then the risk from the amount of x rays delivered to the uterus is very small. Finally, advances in our understanding of the well-being of the fetus by ultrasound, electronic fetal monitors, and even CAT scans certainly can add to the accuracy of the surgical diagnosis without unduly jeopardizing the fetus. In the current environment it is now legitimate to terminate any pregnancy for elective reasons. It would seem worthy of emphasis that there is really very seldom an indication for an abortion, but if the patient wishes to be ultraconservative, then abortion could be offered to her on an elective basis.

INDEX

Abuse drugs, 161
Acromegaly, 37
Acute abdomen, 44
Addison's syndrome, 40
Adrenal cortical deficiency, 40
Adrenal disorders, 38
Adrenal physiology, changes in, 38
Alcohol, 160
Aldosteronism, 39
Amniotic fluid embolization, 30
Analgesics, 151
Androgens, 159
Anesthesia
  management, 7
  maternal, effect on fetus, 4
  perinatal mortality, 6
  premature delivery, 6
  for surgery, 1
  and teratogenicity, 4
Anorectal disease, 57-59
Antibiotics, 28, 152
Anticoagulants, 154
Anticonvulsants, 155
Antidepressants, 159
Antiemetics, 156
Antihypertensives, 157
Antineoplastics, 156
Antipsychotics, 159
Antithyroid drugs, 162
Aorto-caval compression, 2
Appendicitis, 48-50
Arrhythmias, 123

Bladder
  injury in delivery, 74
  and urethra, physiologic changes, 69
Bleeding, gastrointestinal, 45
Blood volume, 3
Bowel obstruction, 50
Breast
  abscess, 105
  adenoma, 106
  benign diseases, 102

Breast (cont'd)
  cancer, 107-116
  chronic cystic mastitis, 103
  chronic suppurative mastitis, 105
  diseases, 101
  ductal papilloma, 105
  ectasia, ductal, 104
  fat necrosis, 104
  feeding and drug effects, 162
  fibroadenoma, 106
  plasma cell mastitis, 104

Cancer
  breast, 107-116
  colon, 61
  stomach, 60
  thyroid, 33
Cardiac arrhythmias, 123
  disease
    acquired, 120
    congenital, 122, 128
Cardiothoracic diseases, 120
Cardiovascular drugs, 157
Cardiovascular physiologic changes,
  2, 27
Cholecystitis, 55
Cirrhosis, hepatic, 59
Colitis, ulcerative, 57
Colon cancer, 61
Congenital urulogic problems, 72
Conn's syndrome, 39
Coronary artery disease, 122
Corticosteroids, 161
Crohn's disease, 55
Cushing's syndrome, 39

Diastasis recti and hernia, 138
Diuretics, 157
Dosage of x-ray exams to ovaries, 15
Drug
  adverse effects, 165-175
  antithyroid, 162
  and breast feeding, 162

Drug (cont'd)
  cardiovascular, 157
  embryonic and fetal development,
     effects on, 150
  gastric pressure, effects on, 3
  nonsteroidal-anti-inflammatory, 152
  psychotropic, 159
  social, 160
  sulfonamides, 153
  teratogenicity, 149
  therapy, 148
  transfer, placental, 149

Embolism, pulmonary, 95, 124
Embolization, amniotic fluid, 30
Endocrine disorders, 32
Enterocolitis, 55
Esophageal hiatus hernia, 53, 125
Estrogens, 158

Fat necrosis, breast, 104
FDA pregnancy drug labeling, 150
Fetal effects of maternal anesthesia,
  4

Galactocele, 105
Gastric cancer, 60
Gastric changes in pregnancy, 3
Gastric pressure, drug effect on, 3
Gastric secretion, 4
Gastroenteric bleeding, 45, 47
Gastroenteric causes, 46
Gastroenteric diseases, 43, 48
  incidence, 44
Gastroenteric physiologic changes, 3

Hazards, x-ray exams, 16
Heart disease
  acquired, 126
  congenital, 122, 128
Hemorrhoids, 58
Hepatic cirrhosis, 59
Hernias, 135
  diaphragmatic, 139
    management in delivery, 140
  diastasis recti, 138
  external, 136
  femoral, 137
  hiatal, 139
  inguinal, 137
  internal, 141
  post-traumatic, 139
  umbilical, 138
  ventral, 138
Hiatus hernia, 125, 139
Hormones, 158

Hyperbaric oxygen, 5
Hyperemesis, 53
Hyperparathyroidism, 35
Hypertension, portal, 59
Hyperthyroidism, 33
Hypoglycemic drugs, 162
Hypoparathyroidism, 36
Hypotension, maternal, 6
Hypothyroidism, 34
Hypoxia, maternal, 5

Injury
  bladder, in delivery, 74
  ureter, in delivery, 75
Infection, urinary tract, 71
Intravenous pyelography, 70
Isotretinoin, 162

Kidney
  abscess, 72
  physiologic changes, 68
  transplant, 76

Leukemia, fetal, after x-ray exams,
  17
Lithium, 160

Mastitis
  chronic
    cystic, 103
    suppurative, 105
  plasma cell, 104
Maternal hypotension, 6
  hypoxia, 5
  physiologic changes, 1
Myasthenia gravis, 125

Narcotics, 151
Neoplasms, urinary tract, 73
Nodular goiter, 33
Nonsteroidal anti-inflammatory drugs,
  152

Obstetrical advances and surgical
  practice, 180

Pancreatitis, 51
Parathyroid disorders, 35
Peptic ulcer, perforation, 47
Pericentesis, 28
Perinatal mortality after anesthesia,
  6
Peripheral vascular physiologic
  changes, 83
Peripheral vascular problems, 82, 94
Phenobarbitol, 156

Phenytoin, 155
Pheochromocytoma, 40
Phlegmasia alba dolens, 91
Phlegmasia cerulea dolens, 92
Physiologic changes, 29
    adrenal, 38
    bladder and urethra, 69
    cardiovascular, 2
    gastrointestinal, 43
    maternal, 1, 29
    parathyroid, 35
    peripheral vascular, 83
    pituitary, 37
    renal, 68, 73
    respiratory, 1, 28
    thyroid, 32
    ureteral, 68
Pituitary adenoma, 38
Pituitary disorders, 37
Placental drug transfer, 149
Portal hypertension, 59
Postpulmonary resection, management, 129
Premature delivery after anesthesia, 6
Psychotropics, 159
Pulmonary disease and surgery, 123
Pulmonary embolism, 95, 124
Pyelography
    intravenous, 70
    retrograde, 70

Renal abscess, 72
Renal scan, 70
Renal transplant, 76
Risk factors in ultrasound exam, 19, 22

Salicylates, 152
Seat belts, 30
Small bowel tumors, 61
Smoking, 160
Social drugs, 160
Sulfonamides, 153
Superficial thrombophlebitis, 89
Surgery
    anesthesia for, 1
    for heart disease, 122
    practice and obstetric advances, 180
    for pulmonary disease, 123
Syncopal syndrome, 2

Teratogenicity
    anesthesia, 4
    drug, 149
Tetracyclines, 153
Thrombophlebitis, superficial, 89
Thrombosis, 87
    deep venous, 89
    venous, disseminated, 92
Thyroid cancer, 33
    disorders, 32
    nodules, 33
    physiologic changes, 32
Transplant, renal, 76
Trauma in pregnancy, 27

Ulcer, peptic, perforation, 47
Ultrasound
    benefits vs risks, 22
    diagnosis, 19
    risk factors, 19, 22
    urologic diagnosis, 70
    usage recommended, 20, 23
Ureter
    injury in labor, 75
    physiologic changes, 68
Urinary stone disease, 73
    tract in pregnancy, 73
        and infection, 71
        injuries, 74
        tumors, 73
Urologic problems, 67
    anatomic considerations, 67
    congenital, 72
    diagnosis, ultrasound, 70
    diseases, 71
    embryonic considerations, 67
    physiologic changes, 68
    x-ray diagnosis, 69
Uterus, rupture, 29

Vaccines in pregnancy, 161
Varicose veins, 86

X-ray examinations, 12, 14
    dosage and ovaries, 15
    hazards of, 16
    and leukemia, 17
    of urologic problems, 69